Timothy P Hu

MW01254464

Handbook of Chronic Myeloid Leukemia

Timothy P Hughes, David M Ross, Junia V Melo

Handbook of Chronic Myeloid Leukemia

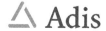 Adis

Timothy P Hughes MD, FRACP, FRCPA, MBBS
SA Pathology & SAHMRI
University of Adelaide
Department of Hematology
Adelaide
Australia

David M Ross MBBS, PhD, FRACP, FRCPA
University of Adelaide and Flinders University
SA Pathology
Department of Hematology
Adelaide
Australia

Junia V Melo MD, PhD, FRCPath
University of Adelaide
Department of Hematology
Adelaide
Australia

ISBN 978-3-319-08349-0   ISBN 978-3-319-08350-6 (eBook)
DOI 10.1007/978-3-319-08350-6
Springer Cham Heidelberg New York Dordrecht London

Printed on acid-free paper

Springer is part of Springer Science+Business Media (www.springer.com)

Project editor: Laura Hajba

Contents

Author biographies

Timothy P Hughes, MD, FRACP, FRCPA, MBBS, is Head of the Department of Hematology at SA Pathology (RAH site) and Head of Translational Leukemia Research at the South Australian Health and Medical Research Institute (SAHMRI). He also holds a Professorial Chair in leukemia research at the University of Adelaide and is a National Health and Medical Research Council (NHMRC) Practitioner Fellow. Professor Hughes' research is focused on studies of the dynamics of response, disease progression, and drug resistance in leukemia. He has published over 250 articles with over 15,000 citations. In 2009 he co-founded the International CML Foundation (iCMLf) with John Goldman and Jorge Cortes and was appointed Chair in 2014.

David M Ross, MBBS, PhD, FRACP, FRCPA, is a Consultant Hematologist in SA Pathology based at the Royal Adelaide Hospital and Flinders Medical Centre in Adelaide, Australia. He undertook his training in clinical and laboratory hematology in Adelaide and Cambridge, UK. He returned to Adelaide to undertake his PhD project on the subject of minimal residual disease in chronic myeloid leukemia (CML) with Tim Hughes, Sue Branford, and Junia Melo. Dr Ross is a member of the disease group for CML and myeloproliferative neoplasms (MPN) in the Australasian Leukemia and Lymphoma Group (ALLG) trials collaborative group. He coordinated the ALLG CML8 clinical trial of imatinib cessation in patients with stable molecular remission (TWISTER). He has been involved in numerous clinical trials in CML and MPN. His current research interests include treatment-free remission in CML and mutations in MPN.

Junia V Melo, MD, PhD, FRCPath, graduated from the Faculty of Medicine, Universidade Federal de Minas Gerais (UFMG), Brazil in 1974, did her internal medicine and hematology training in Rio de Janeiro, Brazil, and earned her PhD from the Royal Postgraduate Medical School (RPMS), University of London in 1986. She did her first post-doctoral training in Adelaide, Australia, after which she was invited to re-join the RPMS as a team leader in the MRC/LRF Adult Leukemia Unit in 1990. She established her research group at Imperial College London & Hammersmith Hospital from 1990 to 2007, as Professor of Molecular Hematology. In 2008 she took up the positions of Head of Leukemia Research at the Division of Hematology, Centre for Cancer Biology, IMVS, Adelaide, and of Professor of Medicine at the University of Adelaide. Her main research is focused on the molecular biology and cell kinetics of chronic myeloid leukemia and related myeloproliferative disorders, and on identifying new molecular targets for the treatment of these diseases. Professor Melo is a member of the Editorial Boards of *Blood*, and *Genes, Chromosomes & Cancer*, of the American Society of Hematology (ASH), and a Fellow of the Royal College of Pathologists, UK (FRCPath). She has authored over 200 publications in peer-reviewed journals.

Abbreviations

ABL	Abelson oncogene
Actin-bind	Actin-binding domain
AKT	AKT8 virus oncogene cellular homolog
ALL	Acute lymphoblastic leukemia
AML	Acute myeloid leukemia
AP	Accelerated phase
BAD	BCL-2 associated death promoter gene
BCR	*Breakpoint cluster region* – gene that fuses with ABL
BCL-2	*B-cell lymphoma-2 gene*
BELA	Bosutinib Efficacy and Safety in Chronic Myeloid Leukemia – Phase III trial of bosutinib versus imatinib
BID	Twice daily
BIM	BCL-2-interacting mediator of cell death
BM	Bone marrow
CBL	Casitas B-lineage lymphoma
CCA	Clonal chromosome abnormalities
CCyR	Complete cytogenetic response
CHR	Complete hematological response
CML	Chronic myeloid leukemia
CMR	Complete molecular response
CRK	*CT10 sarcoma oncogene cellular homolog*
CP	Chronic phase
DASISION	DASatinib versus Imatinib Study In treatment-Naive CML patients
DAS	Dasatinib
DD	Dimerization
DNA-bind	DNA-binding domain
DOK	Downstream of kinase
ELN	European Leukemia Net

ENESTnd	Evaluating Nilotinib Efficacy and Safety in Clinical Trials – Newly Diagnosed Patients
ERK	Extracellular signal-regulated kinase
EUTOS	European Treatment and Outcome Study for CML
FGFR	Fibroblast growth factor receptor
FISH	Fluorescence in situ hybridization
GAP	GTPase-activating protein
G-CSF	Granulocyte-colony stimulating factor
GDP	Guanosine 5′-diphosphate
GM-CSF	Granulocyte-macrophage colony-stimulating factor
GRB-2	Growth factor receptor-bound protein 2
GTP	Guanosine 5′-triphosphate
HSC	Hematopoietic stem cell
IFN	Interferon
IM	Imatinib
IS	International Scale
JAK2	Janus kinase 2
LBC	Lymphoid blast crisis
LDL	Low-density lipoprotein
LGL	Large granular lymphocyte
MAPK	Mitogen-activated protein kinase
MBC	Myeloid blast crisis
MCyR	Major cytogenetic response
MDR	Multi-drug resistance
MEK1/2	MAPK/ERK kinase 1/2
MMR	Major molecular response
MNC	Mononuclear cell
MRD	Minimal residual disease
MYC	Myelocytomatosis oncogene cellular homolog
NA	Non-applicable
NIL	Nilotinib
NLS	Nuclear localization
OCT-1	Organic cation transporter 1

PACE	Ponatinib Ph ALL and CML Evaluation – the Ponatinib Phase II study
PAH	Pulmonary arterial hypertension
PB	Peripheral blood
PCR	Polymerase chain reaction
PCyR	Partial cytogenetic response
Ph	Philadelphia chromosome
PI3K	Phosphatidylinositol 3 kinase
QD	Once daily
RAF-1	*Rapidly accelerated fibrosarcoma gene*
RAS–GAP	Rat sarcoma–GTPase-activating protein
rho-GEF	Rho GTP–GDP exchange factor
RQ-PCR	Real-time quantitive polymerase chain reaction
SAPK	Stress-activated protein kinase
SEQ	Sequence
SH1/2/3	Src-homology 1/2/3
SHC	Src homology 2 domain containing
SOS	Son-of-sevenless
Src	Phospho-serine/threonine rich sequences
STAT	Signal transducer and activator of transcription
STIM	Stop Imatinib – a French trial of imatinib cessation
TFR	Treatment-free remission
TKI	Tyrosine kinase inhibitor
UMRD	Undetectable minimal residual disease

Dedication

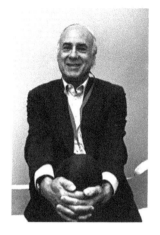

This book is dedicated to our mentor and friend, John M. Goldman. He inspired a generation of hematologists, including all three authors, to follow a career in chronic myeloid leukemia (CML) research.

The authors have donated their writing fees and royalties to support the work of the International CML Foundation (iCMLf), through the 'John Goldman Fund', which will provide training and support for hematologists from developing countries to help them to improve the outcome for their patients with CML.

Chapter 1

Introduction

Chronic myeloid leukemia (CML) is a myeloproliferative disease of the hematopoietic stem cell (HSC). In its natural history, CML is a tri-phasic disease, presenting predominantly in a chronic phase averaging around 5–7 years, but spanning from between a few months to over 20 years. Unless properly treated, the disease progresses through an ill-defined accelerated phase, which leads to transformation into an aggressive acute leukemia or blast crisis. The latter can be of myeloid (approximately 70% of cases) or lymphoid (30%) origin. Until the emergence of tyrosine kinase inhibitors (TKIs), the only curative treatment for CML was HSC transplantation, and this was restricted to a minority of patients, due to age restrictions and the availability of a histocompatible donor. The prognosis has now substantially improved for most CML patients who respond well to TKIs, a proportion of whom remain without evidence of disease even after cessation of treatment.

Historical perspective

The clinical syndrome that we know as CML was first described in the 19th century independently, and virtually simultaneously, by John H Bennett in Scotland and Rudolph Virchow in Germany, based on autopsy observations [1] (Figure 1.1).

The introduction of panoptic blood staining techniques in the 1890s allowed a more precise morphological distinction between granulocytes and lymphocytes and, thus, a better characterization of CML or 'chronic granulocytic leukemia', as a distinct nosological entity.

© Springer International Publishing Switzerland 2014
T.P. Hughes et al., *Handbook of Chronic Myeloid Leukemia*,
DOI 10.1007/978-3-319-08350-6_1

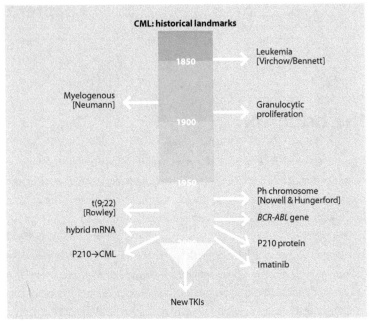

Figure 1.1 Historical landmarks in chronic myeloid leukemia. Historical landmarks which led to our understanding of the biology and clinical features of CML, and which made of CML the paradigm of successful targeted therapy. CML, chronic myeloid leukemia; TKI, tyrosine kinase inhibitor.

The clinical features and evolution of the disease were progressively well documented in the subsequent century. Through a systematic study of 166 patients, Minot and co-workers identified age as a prognostic factor, an observation that has stood the passage of time – age is still a major prognostic factor in the Sokal and Hasford scoring systems [2,3] used nowadays to guide treatment. In 1951, Dameshek made an insightful contribution to the subsequent understanding of the biology of CML, by proposing to include it in the group of myeloproliferative syndromes, together with idiopathic myeloid metaplasia, polycythemia vera, and essential thrombocytosis [4].

In 1960, Nowell and Hungerford reported on the karyotype of seven patients with CML who displayed a small acrocentric G-group chromosome, which resembled the Y chromosome, and named it the Philadelphia (Ph) chromosome [5]. This was a seminal discovery as it was the first consistent cytogenetic abnormality in a human malignancy. The next crucial step in the characterization of this abnormality was made possible by the introduction of G-banding techniques, which allowed Janet Rowley to observe that the Ph chromosome was, in fact, a shortened chromosome 22 (22q-), which was accompanied by another abnormal chromosome, a 9q+, as a result of a reciprocal t(9;22)(q34;q11) translocation [6].

The last quarter of the 20th century brought us, in quick succession, the discoveries which underlie our present knowledge on the molecular biology of CML. These were represented by the isolation of the Abelson (*ABL*) oncogene (*v-ABL*) and its murine (*c-Abl*) and human (*ABL1*) proto-oncogenes [7]; the finding that part of this *ABL* gene translocated to the Ph chromosome [8]; the identification of a 5.8-Kb region of DNA on chromosome 22 where the translocation breakpoints occur, thus termed 'breakpoint cluster region', from which the name of the disrupted gene *BCR* derived [9]; the cloning and sequencing of the actual fusion transcript encrypted by the new *BCR–ABL* hybrid gene formed on the Ph chromosome as a result of the translocation [10–12]; and the discovery that the translated BCR–ABL protein carries abnormal tyrosine kinase activity, which could be important in the pathogenesis of CML [13,14]. This knowledge paved the way for the cornerstone of CML biology – the demonstration that introduction of the *BCR–ABL* gene via a retroviral vector into murine HSCs was capable and sufficient to reproduce a CML-like disease in mice transplanted with these transduced cells [15]. This, in turn, provided the mechanistic basis for the development of targeted therapy for CML in the form of TKIs [16].

Epidemiology

CML has a relatively low incidence of approximately 1–1.5 new cases per 100,000 people per year. However, its prevalence is on the increase due to the significant improvement in its treatment over the past 10 years, enabling patients with CML to achieve survival rates comparable to those of the age-matched healthy population [17]. CML represents 15–20% of all leukemia in adults [18].

In the Western population, the median age of patients at diagnosis is 55–65 years old, with fewer than 10% of cases occurring below the age of 20 years. However, in Asia, Africa, Southern/Eastern Europe, and Latin America the median age of CML is significantly lower, averaging 38–41 years in different countries [19]. The disease affects both sexes, with a slight male preponderance (male:female ratio of 1.3:1).

Etiology

The only known predisposing factor to CML is high-dose ionizing radiation, as best demonstrated by studies of survivors of the Hiroshima and Nagasaki atomic bomb explosions [20]. Apart from a reported borderline increased risk of CML in first-degree relatives of patients with myeloproliferative disorders [21], there is no evidence of an inherited disposition or association with chemical exposure.

Clinical manifestations

Most patients with CML are diagnosed in the chronic phase, which occurs frequently as an incidental finding when blood tests are performed for other reasons. Around one-third of patients are asymptomatic, although other patients typically have mild symptoms of fatigue, weight loss, or sweats [22]. Not uncommonly patients report abdominal discomfort or early satiety due to splenomegaly. Without effective treatment the disease usually transforms to an accelerated phase, which can be associated with increasing leukocytosis and basophilia, splenomegaly, and worsening constitutional symptoms. The average duration of the accelerated phase historically was around 2–3 years, followed by the development of blast crisis. The latter is indistinguishable from acute leukemia with a spectrum of clinical features including leukocytosis, cytopenia, bone pain, and chloroma. Median survival in patients that reached blast crisis and were treated with chemotherapy prior to the advent of TKIs was 3–6 months [23].

Not all patients follow this stepwise progression, and blast crisis can sometimes develop abruptly outside of the chronic phase or be present at diagnosis. Response to therapy and overall survival in advanced phase CML are relatively poor, so the major goal of treatment for chronic phase CML is to prevent progression to the advanced phase.

Pathophysiology

The t(9;22)(q34;q11) reciprocal translocation gives rise to two pathog-nomonic fusion genes, *BCR–ABL* on the 22q- (Ph) chromosome, and *ABL–BCR*, on the derivative 9q+ (Figure 1.2). Although the latter is transcribed, there is no current evidence that it has functional relevance in the disease [24]. Thus, it is the translation of the *BCR–ABL* gene into an abnormal fusion protein that is mostly responsible for the leukemic process.

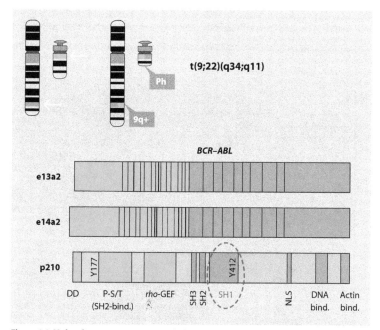

Figure 1.2 Molecular rearrangements underlying chronic myeloid leukemia. Structure of the t(9;22)(q34;q11) reciprocal chromosomal translocation that gives rise to the two derivative chromosomes 9q+ and 22q-, or Ph. The *BCR–ABL* gene is formed on the latter and is transcribed into mRNA with e13a2 or e14a2 junctions. The encoded p210 kD BCR–ABL oncoprotein contains functional domains from the amino-terminus of BCR and the carboxy-terminus of ABL. Shown on the diagram are the dimerization [DD], the phospho-serine/threonine rich sequences within the Src-homology (SH2)-binding (SH2-bind) region, and the *rho* CTP-GDP exchange factor domains (*rho*-GEF) on the BCR part, and the SH3, SH2, and SH1 regions, and the DNA- and actin-binding domains (DNA-bind.; Actin-bind.) on the ABL part. Tyrosine 177 in the Bcr and tyrosine 412 in the Abl regions are important for doscking of adaptor proteins and for BCR–ABL autophosphorylation, respectively. The SH1, encoding the tyrosine kinase domain of the protein, is highlighted by the oval circle. *BCR–ABL*, breakpoint cluster region–Abelson oncogene; NLS, nuclear localization; SH1/2/3, Src-homology 1/2/3; Src, phospho-serine/threonine rich sequences. Reproduced with permission from © Elsevier, 2004. All rights reserved. Melo, Deininger [25].

The BCR–ABL oncoprotein includes several important domains of its parental BCR and ABL normal counterparts, which endow it with specific biological properties (Figure 1.2). The most important feature of this oncoprotein in relation to its leukemogenic action is the fact that the dimerization domain encoded by the amino-terminus of BCR leads to a constitutively activated tyrosine kinase of the ABL portion. As such, BCR–ABL interferes with a series of signal transduction pathways, including the phosphatidylinositol 3 kinase (PI3K), the Janus kinase 2–signal transducer and activator of transcription (JAK2–STAT) and the mitogen-activated protein kinase (MAPK) pathways, among others (Figure 1.3). This leads to exacerbated cell proliferation, decreased adherence to the

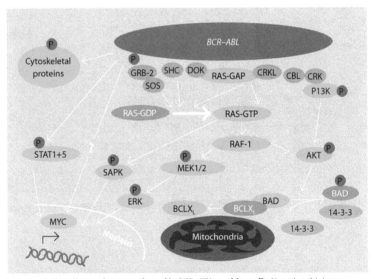

Figure 1.3 Signaling pathways activated in *BCR–ABL*-positive cells. Note that this is a very simplified diagram and that many more associations between BCR–ABL and signaling proteins have been reported. AKT, AKT8 virus oncogene cellular homolog; BAD, BCL-2 associated death promoter gene; BCLXL, B-cell lymphoma XL; *BCR–ABL*, breakpoint cluster region–Abelson oncogene; CBL, Casitas B-lineage lymphoma; CRK, CT10 sarcoma oncogene cellular homolog; DOK, downstream of kinase; ERK, extracellular signal-regulated kinase; GAP, GTPase-activating protein; GDP, guanosine 5'-diphosphate; GRB-2, growth factor receptor-bound protein 2; GTP, guanosine 5'-triphosphate; MAPK, mitogen-activated protein kinase; MEK1/2, MAPK/ERK kinase 1/2; MYC, myelocytomatosis oncogene cellular homolog; PI3K, phosphatidylinositol 3 kinase; RAF-1, rapidly accelerated fibrosarcoma gene; SAPK, stress-activated protein kinase; SHC, Src homology 2 domain containing; SOS , son-of-sevenless; STAT1+5, signal transducer and activator of transcription 1+5. Reproduced with permission from © American Society of Hemtology, 2000. All rights reserved. Deininger et al [26].

bone marrow stroma, reduced response to apoptotic stimuli, and increased genomic instability [26]. These basic biological changes are responsible for the cellular phenotype of chronic phase CML, and pave the way for disease transformation.

The genetic event that triggers CML, or the t(9;22) translocation, occurs in a pluripotent HSC and is, therefore, found in nearly all the derived cell lineages, in spite of the predominant neutrophilic leukocytosis and thrombocytosis. During the chronic phase, there is a significant expansion of the myeloid progenitors, which still have a nearly intact capacity to differentiate, mature, and function properly. However, with progression of the disease due to the acquisition of additional cytogenetic and genetic abnormalities, the leukemic clone undergoes differentiation arrest, resulting in a major increase of immature blasts at the expense of the terminally differentiated leucocytes [27]. The biological process behind this transformation is reported to be a change in character of the granulocyte-macrophage progenitors which, due to abnormal b-catenin signaling, acquire the stem cell-like capacity of unrestricted self-renewal and, thus, repopulate the bone marrow with immature cells [28].

References

1   Piller G. Leukaemia—a brief historical review from ancient times to 1950. *Br J Haematol.* 2001;112:282-29.
2   Sokal JE, Cox EB, Baccarani M, et al. Prognostic discrimination in «good-risk» chronic granulocytic leukemia. *Blood.* 1984;63:789-799.
3   Hasford J, Pfirrmann M, Hehlmann R, et al. A new prognostic score for survival of patients with chronic myeloid leukemia treated with interferon alfa. Writing Committee for the Collaborative CML Prognostic Factors Project Group. *J Natl Cancer Inst.* 1998;90:850-858.
4   Damesek W. Some speculations on the myeloproliferative syndromes. *Blood.* 1951;6:372-375.
5   Nowell PC, Hungerford DA. A minute chromosome in human chronic granulocytic leukemia. *Science.* 1960;132:1497.
6   Rowley JD. A new consistent chromosomal abnormality in chronic myelogenous leukaemia identified by quinacrine fluorescence and Giemsa staining. *Nature.* 1973;243:290-293.
7   Goff SP, Gilboa E, Witte ON, Baltimore D. Structure of the Abelson murine leukemia virus genome and the homologous cellular gene: studies with cloned viral DNA. *Cell.* 1980;22:777-785.
8   de KA, van Kessel AG, Grosveld G, et al. A cellular oncogene is translocated to the Philadelphia chromosome in chronic myelocytic leukaemia. *Nature.* 1982;300:765-767.
9   Groffen J, Stephenson JR, Heisterkamp N, de Klein A, Bartram CR, Grosveld G. Philadelphia chromosomal breakpoints are clustered within a limited region, bcr, on chromosome 22. *Cell.* 1984;36:93-99.
10 Canaani E, Gale RP, Steiner Saltz D, Berrebi A, Aghai E, Januszewicz E. Altered transcription of an oncogene in chronic myeloid leukaemia. *Lancet.* 1984;1:593-595.

11   Shtivelman E, Lifshitz B, Gale RP, Canaani E. Fused transcript of abl and bcr genes in chronic myelogenous leukaemia. *Nature*. 1985;315:550-554.

12   Grosveld G, Verwoerd T, van AT, et al. The chronic myelocytic cell line K562 contains a breakpoint in bcr and produces a chimeric bcr/c-abl transcript. *Mol Cell Biol*. 1986;6:607-616.

13   Konopka JB, Watanabe SM, Witte ON. An alteration of the human c-abl protein in K562 leukemia cells unmasks associated tyrosine kinase activity. *Cell*. 1984;37:1035-1042.

14   Ben Neriah Y, Bernards A, Paskind M, Daley GQ, Baltimore D. Alternative 5' exons in c-abl mRNA. *Cell*. 1986; 44:577-586.

15   Daley GQ, Van Etten RA, Baltimore D. Induction of chronic myelogenous leukemia in mice by the P210bcr/abl gene of the Philadelphia chromosome. *Science*. 1990;247:824-830.

16   Druker BJ. Translation of the Philadelphia chromosome into therapy for CML. *Blood*. 2008; 112:4808-4817.

17   Hoglund M, Sandin F, Hellstrom K, et al. Tyrosine kinase inhibitor usage, treatment outcome, and prognostic scores in CML: report from the population-based Swedish CML registry. *Blood*. 2013;122:1284-1292.

18   Siegel R, Naishadham D, Jemal A. Cancer statistics, 2012. *CA Cancer J Clin*. 2012;62:10-29.

19   Mendizabal AM, Garcia-Gonzalez P, Levine PH. Regional variations in age at diagnosis and overall survival among patients with chronic myeloid leukemia from low and middle income countries. *Cancer Epidemiol*. 2013;37:247-254.

20   Bizzozero OJ, Jr, Johnson KG, Ciocco A. Radiation-related leukemia in Hiroshima and Nagasaki, 1946–1964. I. Distribution, incidence and appearance time. *N Engl J Med*. 1966;274:1095-1101.

21   Landgren O, Goldin LR, Kristinsson SY, Helgadottir EA, Samuelsson J, Bjorkholm M. Increased risks of polycythemia vera, essential thrombocythemia, and myelofibrosis among 24,577 first-degree relatives of 11,039 patients with myeloproliferative neoplasms in Sweden. *Blood*. 2008;112:2199-2204.

22   Hehlmann R, Heimpel H, Hasford J, et al. Randomized comparison of busulfan and hydroxyurea in chronic myelogenous leukemia: prolongation of survival by hydroxyurea. The German CML Study Group. *Blood*. 1993;82:398-407.

23   Sacchi S, Kantarjian HM, O'Brien S, et al. Chronic myelogenous leukemia in nonlymphoid blastic phase: analysis of the results of first salvage therapy with three different treatment approaches for 162 patients. *Cancer*. 1999;86:2632-2641.

24   Melo JV, Gordon DE, Cross NC, Goldman JM. The ABL-BCR fusion gene is expressed in chronic myeloid leukemia. *Blood*. 1993;81:158-165.

25   Melo J, Deininger MW. Biology of chronic myelogenous leukemia—signaling pathways of initiation and transformation. *Hematol Oncol Clin North Am*. 2004;18:545-568.

26   Deininger MW, Goldman JM, Melo JV. The molecular biology of chronic myeloid leukemia. *Blood*. 2000;96:3343-3356.

27   Melo JV, Barnes DJ. Chronic myeloid leukaemia as a model of disease evolution in human cancer. *Nat Rev Cancer*. 2007;7:441-453.

28   Jamieson CH, Ailles LE, Dylla SJ, et al. Granulocyte-macrophage progenitors as candidate leukemic stem cells in blast-crisis CML. *N Engl J Med*. 2004;351:657-667.

Chapter 2

Diagnosis

When a patient presents with suspected chronic myeloid leukemia (CML) appropriate assessments are needed to confirm the diagnosis and stage of disease, and to assign a risk score to that patient.

Diagnostic laboratory tests

Blood picture and biochemistry

Most chronic phase CML patients present with a characteristic blood picture with increased and left-shifted granulopoiesis, and a predominance of neutrophils and myelocytes (Figure 2.1). There is also an increase in eosinophils and basophils.

A variant presentation of chronic phase CML is marked thrombocytosis with little or no neutrophilia, mimicking essential thrombocythemia. Another rare presentation mimics chronic myelomonocytic leukemia with predominant monocytosis: such cases may express p190 breakpoint cluster region–Abelson (*BCR–ABL*) oncogene [1]. Biochemical correlates of myeloid hyperplasia include increased uric acid and lactate dehydrogenase.

Bone marrow morphology

The bone marrow is markedly hypercellular with granulocytic and variable megakaryocytic hyperplasia, and relatively depressed erythropoiesis (Figures 2.2 and 2.3).

The differential counts resemble those in the peripheral blood with left-shift eosinophilia and basophilia. The megakaryocytes have

© Springer International Publishing Switzerland 2014
T.P. Hughes et al., *Handbook of Chronic Myeloid Leukemia*,
DOI 10.1007/978-3-319-08350-6_2

a typical morphology with a marked increase in small, hypolobated forms. Dysplastic features are unusual. The cytoplasm of debris-laden macrophages can have a characteristic deep blue (sea blue histiocytes) or crinkled tissue paper appearance (pseudo-Gaucher cells), reflecting increased cell turnover. Reticulin fibrosis is not usually seen, but a minority of CML cases can have significant fibrosis, resulting in features that may resemble primary myelofibrosis. The presence of marrow fibrosis in CML has been reported as an adverse prognostic factor, and can be associated with disease progression [2].

The blast crisis bone marrow shows features that would be expected in de novo acute myeloid leukemia (AML) or acute lymphoblastic leukemia (ALL), but there may be morphological clues to the origin of the leukemia, such as eosinophilia or basophilia. In the accelerated phase there are features intermediate between the chronic and blast crisis phases. Diagnostic criteria for CML disease phase are summarized in Table 2.1.

The criteria of Kantarjian and colleagues have been widely used in clinical trials [3]. Accelerated phase CML can be defined solely on the basis of karyotypic clonal evolution, with blood and marrow morphology

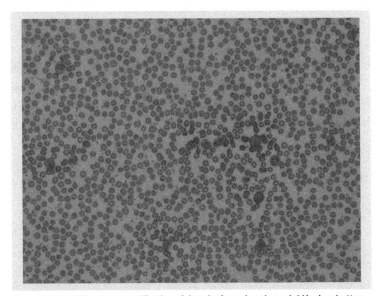

Figure 2.1 Blood film x200 magnification of chronic phase chronic myeloid leukemia. Note the bimodal differential count with peaks in the neutrophils and myelocytes.

consistent with ongoing chronic phase. Accelerated phase patients, defined solely by cytogenetic clonal evolution, may have a better prognosis than those with hematological acceleration [4,5].

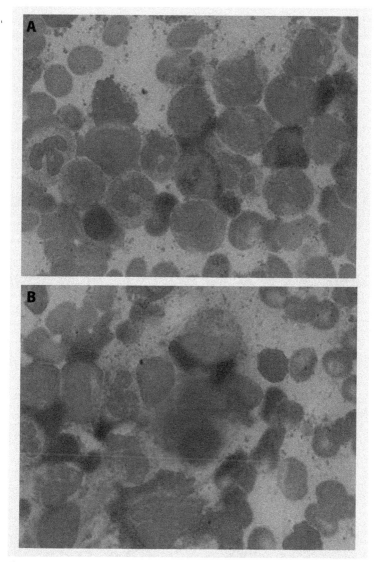

Figure 2.2 Bone marrow aspirate x1000 magnification of chronic phase chronic myeloid leukemia. Note **A,** the prominent eosinophils and **B,** micromegakaryocyte.

Immunophenotyping

Immunophenotyping is not required to diagnose CML in the chronic or accelerated phase. In blast crisis the immunophenotype is helpful in confirming the lineage of the leukemia, which is myeloid in approximately two-thirds of cases and B-lymphoid in approximately one-third of cases; cases with a T-cell lineage are rare. Aberrant expression of lineage-associated markers is commonly observed, and biphenotypic leukemia is seen in a small proportion of cases [6,7].

Cytogenetics

CML is associated with the classical Philadelphia (Ph) chromosome, an abnormally shortened chromosome 22 due to t(9;22)(q22;q34) seen on G-banded karyotypic examination in at least 90–95% of cases (Figure 2.4).

A variant Ph-rearrangement, often involving other chromosomes in addition to chromosomes 9 and 22, may be identified in a further 5% of cases. A cytogenetically cryptic Ph rearrangement is observed in rare

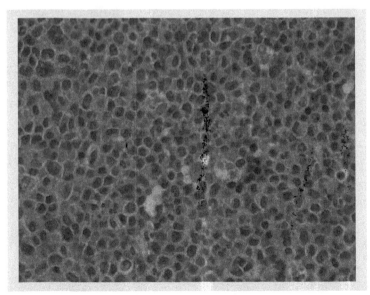

Figure 2.3 **Bone marrow trephine.** Note the near-complete obliteration of fat spaces and proliferation of granulocyte and megakaryocyte lineages. Micromegakaryocytes and debris-laden macrophages can be seen.

	Chronic phase All of the following		Accelerated phase Any of the following		Blast crisis Any of the following	
	WHO [8]	Kantarjian [3]	WHO [8]	Kantarjian [3]	WHO [8]	Kantarjian [3]
Blasts in either PB or BM (%)	<10	<15	10–19	15–29	≥20	≥30
Blasts + promyelocytes in either PB or BM (%)	NR [3]	<30	NR	≥30	NR	NR
Basophils in PB (%)	<20	<20	≥20	≥20	NR	NR
Platelet count (x 10^9/L)	≥100 & ≤1000	≥100	<100 unrelated to therapy or >1000 unresponsive to therapy	<100 unrelated to therapy	NR	NR
WHO classification only						
Increasing spleen size and/or leukocytosis unresponsive to therapy	Absent		Present		NR	
Acquired cytogenetic clonal evolution	Absent		Present		NR	
Extramedullary or focal BM blast proliferation (chloroma)	Absent		Absent		Present	

Table 2.1 Criteria for disease phase in chronic myeloid leukemia. BM, bone marrow; NR, not required; PB, peripheral blood; WHO, World Health Organization. Reproduced with permission from © Wiley, 1988. All rights reserved. Kantarjian et al [3]. Reproduced with permission from © IARC, 2008. All rights reserved. Swerdlow et al [8].

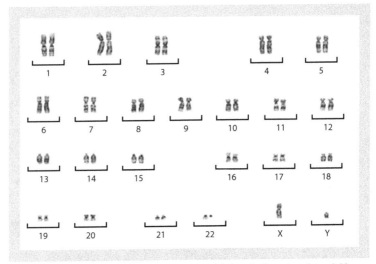

Figure 2.4 Metaphase karyotype of a male patient with chronic phase chronic myeloid leukemia. One long arm of chromosome 9 contains additional material derived from one of the long arms of chromosome 22, resulting in the shortened Philadelphia chromosome. *BCR–ABL* is formed on chromosome 22 and the reciprocal *ABL–BCR* gene is formed on chromosome 9.

cases, which can be detected only by fluorescence in situ hybridization (FISH) or polymerase chain reaction (PCR) [8]. Variant Ph rearrangements do not seem to influence prognosis in patients treated with imatinib [9,10].

In addition to the Ph rearrangement, other chromosomal abnormalities can be observed at diagnosis in around 10% of patients [11]. Selected high-risk additional chromosomal abnormalities (Ph duplication, isochromosome 17q, and trisomy 8) are referred to as 'major route' abnormalities and are associated with a significantly inferior response to treatment [10]. Other additional chromosomal abnormalities (including loss of the Y chromosome) do not seem to have an influence on prognosis.

Molecular studies

Qualitative reverse transcriptase (RT)-PCR for *BCR–ABL* can be used to confirm the presence of the translocation and this method may be the only means of confirming a molecular diagnosis in cases with a cryptic Ph rearrangement. The use of long template PCR with a forward primer in *BCR* exon 1 and a reverse primer in *ABL1* exon 3 enables the detection of not only the typical e13a2 and e14a2 *BCR–ABL* transcripts, but also rarer *BCR–ABL* variants, such as e1a2 (p190 *BCR–ABL*) and e19a2 (p230 *BCR–ABL*), which may otherwise cause diagnostic difficulties [12]. A multiplex RT-PCR assay has been widely used and incorporates primers for e13a2, e14a2 and e1a2 [13]. It is important to be aware of what method is being used in the laboratory in order to be certain that the rarer molecular variants of *BCR–ABL* have been excluded.

The typical p210 BCR–ABL protein that is expressed in CML can be associated with either e13a2 or e14a2 mRNA transcripts. The majority of patients (~60%) express e14a2 only and ~30% of patients express e13a2 only [14–16]; the remainder express both transcripts because of the presence of a polymorphic splice acceptor site that results in splicing out of the 75 bases of *BCR* exon 14 and, consequently, a proportion of the e14a2 being processed to e13a2 [17,18]. While some authors have reported prognostic relevance of the transcript type, there is no convincing evidence of a difference in outcome between patients with p210 CML according to *BCR* breakpoint and mRNA transcript type [15,16,19].

In rare cases, Ph-positive patients express an e19a2 *BCR–ABL* mRNA transcript that results in a p230 BCR–ABL protein. In comparison with classical CML, the resulting syndrome of neutrophilic CML is character-ized by less marked leukocytosis, frequent thrombocytosis, the absence of splenomegaly, and a more indolent disease course [20]. However, clonal evolution can be associated with acceleration in patients with neutrophilic CML, and progression to blast crisis may occur. It is impor-tant to distinguish between neutrophilic CML and chronic neutrophilic leukemia, a rare *BCR–ABL*-negative myeloproliferative syndrome with prominent neutrophilia and hepatosplenomegaly, which, in around half of cases, is associated with activating mutations in the receptor for colony-stimulating factor 3, and which may be sensitive to SRC or Janus kinase (JAK) inhibition [21].

Differential diagnosis

In most cases the diagnosis of CML is uncomplicated, with a typical blood picture and confirmatory cytogenetic or molecular tests. Other hemato-logical malignancies and reactive conditions have features that overlap with CML, and some conditions that may mimic CML are discussed here.

Reactive conditions

'Leukemoid reaction' is a term that is used to describe reactive leukocytosis with predominant neutrophilia that may resemble CML. Cytochemical staining for neutrophil alkaline phosphatase was used to distinguish between leukemoid reaction and CML, but is now obsolete where PCR for *BCR–ABL* is readily available. Immune-mediated disorders such as vasculitis, allergy, and parasitic infection may cause leukocytosis with eosinophilia, but are rarely confused with CML.

Other hematological neoplasms

Chronic Ph-negative myeloproliferative neoplasms such as primary myelofibrosis may present with leukocytosis with eosinophilia or splenomegaly, as may rare cases of myelodysplasia, or the myelodysplastic and myeloproliferative overlap syndromes. Chronic myeloproliferative neoplasms associated with tyrosine kinase fusion genes other than *BCR–ABL* may resemble CML, but are usually evident on karyotyping. These include *ETV6–ABL* with t(9;12), *ETV6–PDGFRB* with t(5;12), and fibroblast growth factor receptor (FGFR) fusions with abnormalities of chromosome 8p. Chronic eosinophilic leukemia with the *FIP1L1–PDGFRA* fusion is cytogenetically cryptic, and can be identified only by FISH or PCR [22].

Eosinophilia and splenomegaly may occur in lymphoproliferative conditions (especially Hodgkin lymphoma and T-cell lymphoma) in which eosinophilia is thought to be driven by abnormal production of cytokines such as interleukin 3 (IL-3), IL-5, and granulocyte-macrophage colony-stimulating factor (GM-CSF) related to the lymphoid clone [8]. Acute leukemia may mimic blast crisis CML, particularly in conditions such as AML with eosinophilia (eg inv[16]), and AML with basophilia (eg t[6;9]). Clinical features and karyotyping may not reliably distinguish between lymphoid blast crisis CML and Ph-positive ALL if there is no prior history of CML.

Clinical risk scores

Clinical risk scores were developed in the 1980s and 1990s, driven by the availability of allogeneic stem cell transplantation as a potentially curative treatment for CML patients. For example, Sokal and colleagues [23] developed a scoring system that divided patients with CML into three risk groups: high (median survival 32 months), intermediate (median survival approximately 45 months), and low (median survival 60 months). This enabled the selection of patients for whom the risk–benefit ratio of the allograft procedure was most favorable. The Sokal score is calculated at diagnosis from the age of the patient, palpable spleen size (in centimeters below the costal margin), platelet count, and blast percentage in the peripheral blood. Elements of the Sokal score overlap with those that are used to define the accelerated phase, so that there is a continuum between high-risk chronic phase and accelerated phase disease, and the definitions that are used to classify patients are somewhat arbitrary. The Sokal score was developed for patients treated with hydroxyurea or busulphan but it is also useful for predicting the outcome for patients treated with imatinib de novo [24,25].

Other scoring systems have been used, including the Hasford score, which was developed in interferon-treated patients. This score incorporates the same four variables as the Sokal score, in addition to the eosinophil count and basophil count in the peripheral blood at the time of diagnosis [26,27]. The more recent European Treatment and Outcome Study for CML (EUTOS) score was developed in imatinib-treated patients and uses only the spleen size and percentage of basophils in the peripheral blood [28]. In an independent series of over 1000 patients this score was predictive of progression-free and overall survival, but not all studies have confirmed these findings [29,30].

References

1 Melo JV, Myint H, Galton DA, Goldman JM. P190BCR-ABL chronic myeloid leukaemia: the missing link with chronic myelomonocytic leukaemia? *Leukemia*. 1994;8:208-211.
2 Buesche G, Ganser A, Schlegelberger B, et al. Marrow fibrosis and its relevance during imatinib treatment of chronic myeloid leukemia. *Leukemia*. 2007;21:2420-2427.
3 Kantarjian HM, Dixon D, Keating MJ, et al. Characteristics of accelerated disease in chronic myelogenous leukemia. *Cancer*. 1988;61:1441-1446.
4 Cortes JE, Talpaz M, Giles F, et al. Prognostic significance of cytogenetic clonal evolution in patients with chronic myelogenous leukemia on imatinib mesylate therapy. *Blood*. 2003;101:3794-3800.
5 O'Dwyer ME, Mauro MJ, Kurilik G, et al. The impact of clonal evolution on response to imatinib mesylate (STI571) in accelerated phase CML. *Blood*. 2002;100:1628-1633.
6 Saikia T, Advani S, Dasgupta A, et al. Characterisation of blast cells during blastic phase of chronic myeloid leukaemia by immunophenotyping--experience in 60 patients. *Leuk Res*. 1988;12:499-506.

7   Khalidi HS, Brynes RK, Medeiros LJ, et al. The immunophenotype of blast transformation of chronic myelogenous leukemia: a high frequency of mixed lineage phenotype in "lymphoid" blasts and A comparison of morphologic, immunophenotypic, and molecular findings. *Mod Pathol.* 1998;11:1211-1221.

8   Swerdlow S, Campo W, Harris N, et al, eds. *WHO Classification of Tumours of Haematopoeitic and Lymphoid Tissues.* Lyon: IARC; 2008.

9   Marzocchi G, Castagnetti F, Luatti S, et al. Variant Philadelphia translocations: molecular-cytogenetic characterization and prognostic influence on frontline imatinib therapy, a GIMEMA Working Party on CML analysis. *Blood.* 2011;117:6793-6800.

10   Fabarius A, Leitner A, Hochhaus A, et al. Impact of additional cytogenetic aberrations at diagnosis on prognosis of CML: long-term observation of 1151 patients from the randomized CML Study IV. *Blood.* 2011;118:6760-6768.

11   O'Brien SG, Guilhot F, Larson RA, et al. Imatinib compared with interferon and low-dose cytarabine for newly diagnosed chronic-phase chronic myeloid leukemia. *N Engl J Med.* 2003;348:994-1004.

12   Branford S, Hughes TP. Diagnosis and monitoring of chronic myeloid leukemia by qualitative and quantitative RT-PCR. In: Iland HJ, Hertzberg M, Marlton P, eds. *Myeloid Leukemia: Methods and Protocols, Methods in Molecular Medicine.* Totawa, NJ: Humana Press; 2006:69-92.

13   Cross NC, Melo JV, Feng L, Goldman JM. An optimized multiplex polymerase chain reaction (PCR) for detection of BCR-ABL fusion mRNAs in haematological disorders. *Leukemia.* 1994;8:186-189.

14   de la Fuente J, Merx K, Steer EJ, et al. ABL-BCR expression does not correlate with deletions on the derivative chromosome 9 or survival in chronic myeloid leukemia. *Blood.* 2001;98:2879-2880.

15   Rozman C, Urbano-Ispizua A, Cervantes F, et al. Analysis of the clinical relevance of the breakpoint location within M-BCR and the type of chimeric mRNA in chronic myelogenous leukemia. *Leukemia.* 1995;9:1104-1107.

16   Shepherd P, Suffolk R, Halsey J, Allan N. Analysis of molecular breakpoint and m-RNA transcripts in a prospective randomized trial of interferon in chronic myeloid leukaemia: no correlation with clinical features, cytogenetic response, duration of chronic phase, or survival. *Br J Haematol.* 1995;89:546-554.

17   Saussele S, Weisser A, Müller MC, et al. Frequent polymorphism in BCR exon b2 identified in BCR-ABL positive and negative individuals using fluorescent hybridization probes. *Leukemia.* 2000;14:2006-2010.

18   Branford S, Hughes TP, Rudzki Z. Dual transcription of b2a2 and b3a2 BCR-ABL transcripts in chronic myeloid leukaemia is confined to patients with a linked polymorphism within the BCR gene. *Br J Haematol.* 2002;117:875-877.

19   Morris SW, Daniel L, Ahmed CM, Elias A, Lebowitz P. Relationship of bcr breakpoint to chronic phase duration, survival, and blast crisis lineage in chronic myelogenous leukemia patients presenting in early chronic phase. *Blood.* 1990;75:2035-2041.

20   Pane F, Intrieri M, Quintarelli C, Izzo B, Muccioli GC, Salvatore F. *BCR/ABL* genes and leukemic phenotype: from molecular mechanisms to clinical correlations. *Oncogene.* 2002;21:8652-8667.

21   Maxson JE, Gotlib J, Pollyea DA, et al. Oncogenic CSF3R mutations in chronic neutrophilic leukemia and atypical CML. *N Engl J Med.* 2013;368:1781-1790.

22   Cools J, DeAngelo DJ, Gotlib J, et al. A tyrosine kinase created by fusion of the *PDGFRA* and *FIP1L1* genes as a therapeutic target of imatinib in idiopathic hypereosinophilic syndrome. *N Engl J Med.* 2003;348:1201-1214.

23   Sokal JE, Cox EB, Baccarani M, et al. Prognostic discrimination in «good-risk» chronic granulocytic leukemia. *Blood.* 1984;63:789-799.

24 Hughes TP, Kaeda J, Branford S, et al. Frequency of major molecular responses to imatinib or interferon alfa plus cytarabine in newly diagnosed chronic myeloid leukemia. *N Engl J Med*. 2003;349:1423-1432.

25 Druker BJ, Guilhot F, O'Brien SG, et al. Five-year follow-up of patients receiving imatinib for chronic myeloid leukemia. *N Engl J Med*. 2006;355:2408-2417.

26 Kantarjian HM, Smith TL, McCredie KB, et al. Chronic myelogenous leukemia: a multivariate analysis of the associations of patient characteristics and therapy with survival. *Blood*. 1985;66:1326-1335.

27 Hasford J, Pfirrmann M, Hehlmann R, et al. A new prognostic score for survival of patients with chronic myeloid leukemia treated with interferon alfa. Writing Committee for the Collaborative CML Prognostic Factors Project Group. *J Natl Cancer Inst*. 1998;90:850-858.

28 Hasford J, Baccarani M, Hoffmann V, et al. Predicting complete cytogenetic response and subsequent progression-free survival in 2060 patients with CML on imatinib treatment: the EUTOS score. *Blood*. 2011;118:686-692.

29 Hoffmann VS, Baccarani M, Lindoerfer D, et al. The EUTOS prognostic score: review and validation in 1288 patients with CML treated frontline with imatinib. *Leukemia*. 2013;27:2016-2022.

30 Jabbour E, Cortes J, Nazha A, et al. EUTOS score is not predictive for survival and outcome in patients with early chronic phase chronic myeloid leukemia treated with tyrosine kinase inhibitors: a single institution experience. *Blood*. 2012;119:4524-4526.

Chapter 3

Monitoring response to treatment

A reduction in the number of leukemic cells in chronic myeloid leukemia (CML) is associated with improved progression-free survival. The careful monitoring of response to treatment is essential to ensure that a patient is on track to achieve long-term disease control. Treatment goals for CML are the normalization of peripheral blood counts, the reduction and elimination of the Philadelphia (Ph) chromosome, and the reduction and elimination of *BCR–ABL* gene expression. Progress toward these goals can be monitored by measuring hematologic, cytogenetic, and molecular responses, respectively (Table 3.1). Monitoring response to therapy for patients with CML is fundamental for achieving optimal patient outcomes and regularly scheduled monitoring after treatment initiation may help identify patients at risk of treatment failure.

Hematological response

The criteria for a complete hematological response (CHR) are detailed in Table 3.1. Normalization of the blood counts and resolution of splenomegaly is typically seen within the first weeks of tyrosine kinase inhibitor (TKI) treatment for chronic phase CML. Its utility for the monitoring of chronic phase CML beyond that time is limited.

Cytogenetic response

Examination of at least 20 bone marrow metaphases was for many years the 'gold standard' for response to treatment in CML. Criteria for different levels of cytogenetic response are defined in Table 3.1. Cytogenetic

© Springer International Publishing Switzerland 2014
T.P. Hughes et al., *Handbook of Chronic Myeloid Leukemia*,
DOI 10.1007/978-3-319-08350-6_3

Hematologic and cytogenetic response definitions in chronic myeloid leukemia	
Complete hematologic response	All of the following:
	Normalization of peripheral blood counts
	Normal white cell differential (no peripheral blood blasts and promyelocytes, sum of myelocytes + metamyelocytes <5%)
	No disease-related symptoms or extramedullary disease, including hepatosplenomegaly
Cytogenetic responses	Defined according to percentage of Ph+ metaphases in bone marrow:
	Minimal >65–95% Ph+
	Minor >35–65%
	Partial >0–35%
	Complete 0%
Major cytogenetic response	Partial or complete cytogenetic response
	≤35% Ph-positive cells detected in a bone marrow sample with a minimum of 20 metaphases
	Approximately equivalent to BCR–ABL <10%
Complete cytogenetic response	0% Ph-positive cells detected in a bone marrow sample with a minimum of 20 metaphases
	Approximately equivalent to BCR–ABL <1%

Table 3.1 Hematologic and cytogenetic response definitions in chronic myeloid leukemia. BCR–ABL, breakpoint cluster region–Abelson oncogene; Ph, Philadelphia chromosome.

response is associated with reduced rates of progression to advanced phase disease, and prolonged overall survival [1–3]. Cytogenetic evolution in the Ph-positive clone is associated with advanced phase disease and a poor prognosis [4–6]. The emergence of clonal evolution during treatment is strongly associated with loss of response [7,8], and presumably reflects inadequate suppression of the genetically unstable CML clone.

Bone marrow cytogenetic monitoring has several limitations for long-term monitoring. Bone marrow aspiration is an invasive procedure with small, but significant, risks attached [9,10]. At least 5% of marrow aspirate samples will yield fewer than 20 metaphases of suitable quality for cytogenetic examination [11,12]. Interphase fluorescence in situ hybridization (FISH) analysis using BCR–ABL-specific probes enables the examination of a greater number of cells, and may therefore provide a more reliable measure of disease burden [13], but real-time quantitive polymerase chain reaction (RQ-PCR) has largely supplanted cytogenetic approaches for quantification of disease burden.

Karyotyping may rarely provide clinically important information on acquired cytogenetic abnormalities in Ph-negative cells during treatment. Around 5% of patients will develop cytogenetic abnormalities in Ph-negative cells during imatinib treatment. These abnormalities might be pre-existing subclones that are revealed by suppression of the CML clone, rather than a consequence of TKI toxicity. These Ph-negative clones have rarely been associated with cytopenia, myelodysplasia, or secondary acute myeloid leukaemia (AML) [14–17]. In the absence of cytopenia or dysplastic changes in the blood there is little to be gained by regular cytogenetic screening of the marrow to identify or monitor these abnormal Ph-negative clones in patients who achieve and maintain satisfactory molecular responses.

Molecular monitoring methods

RQ-PCR detection of *BCR–ABL* forms the backbone of CML monitoring in many centers around the world. RNA is extracted from peripheral blood or bone marrow cells and amplified by using a reverse transcriptase enzyme and either random oligonucleotide primers or sequence-specific primers. An aliquot of the cDNA product is then used in RQ-PCR to quantify both the target transcript *BCR–ABL* and a control gene transcript. The RQ-PCR result is expressed as a ratio of *BCR–ABL* to its control gene.

Several different control genes have been used for *BCR–ABL* RQ-PCR, but the ideal control gene should have expression levels and degradation characteristics similar to *BCR–ABL*, and should be stable in its expression regardless of the disease state and treatment [18,19]. The Europe Against Cancer collaborative group [19] has recommended the use of the control genes *ABL, BCR,* or *GUSB. ABL* is somewhat problematic early in treatment, since both *BCR–ABL* and *ABL* are measured, resulting in a lower *BCR–ABL*/control gene ratio. As the level of residual disease falls the relative contribution of *BCR–ABL* to total *ABL* becomes irrelevant, and all three control genes give similar results with *BCR–ABL* <10%.

Considerable effort has been made to standardize RQ-PCR procedures in a manner similar to that undertaken decades ago to establish the International Normalized Ratio for warfarin therapy [20,21]. Standardized laboratories report *BCR–ABL* on the International Scale. This system was developed following the exchange of clinical trial samples between three reference laboratories [22], which have subsequently undertaken sample exchange with multiple other laboratories around the world. A three-log reduction in *BCR–ABL* from the standardized median baseline level was assigned a value of 0.1% *BCR–ABL*^IS and all other values are determined relative to this set point [23,24]. A value of ≤0.1% is a major molecular response (MMR). The median *BCR–ABL* value at diagnosis in any standardized lab will be close to 100%, but the actual value may vary significantly in an individual patient. An international reference material for *BCR–ABL* was recently synthesized and validated [25]. The use of commercial calibrators and standards should greatly simplify the *BCR–ABL* standardization process.

A simplified approach to standardization is provided by the Cepheid GeneXpert(R) system, an automated sample preparation and real-time PCR detection system [26]. This proprietary tool uses a point-of-care style cartridge that requires minimal training and quality assurance procedures for the end-user. Whole blood is injected into the cartridge and the RQ-PCR is performed in a closed system. Each batch of cartridges is assigned *BCR–ABL*^IS conversion factors by the manufacturer [26].

Molecular response as a surrogate for cytogenetics

Molecular surrogates for cytogenetic response have been reported by several groups, and are now commonly used in clinical practice (Figure 3.1).

The United States National Comprehensive Cancer Network guidelines now refer to molecular response targets [27]. 10% *BCR–ABL* is approximately equivalent to major cytogenetic response (MCyR), while 1% *BCR–ABL* is approximately equivalent to complete cytogenetic response (CCyR) [11,15,28,29]. In 320 samples where RQ-PCR and bone marrow karyotype were performed at the same time point every patient in MMR was also in CCyR [15]. For patients in MMR bone marrow aspiration provides little or no additional information about the Ph-positive clone.

Early molecular response

Several studies have shown that the *BCR–ABL* level achieved following 3 months of TKI treatment is associated with longer term treatment outcomes [30–32]. A *BCR–ABL* value of ≤10% at 3 months is associated

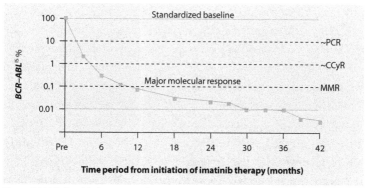

Figure 3.1 Relationship between molecular and cytogenetic response levels. *BCR–ABL*^{IS}, breakpoint cluster region–Abelson oncogene; CCyR, complete cytogenetic response; MMR, major molecular response; PCR, partial cytogenetic response.

with superior rates of MMR and deeper molecular responses, and in some studies with improved progression-free and overall survival. On average this early molecular response target represents a one-log reduction from baseline; however there is significant variation in the *BCR–ABL* level at diagnosis, and the predictive value of the 10% target at 3 months can be improved by an assessment of the drop from the individual baseline value of the patient [33,34].

Undetectable *BCR–ABL* and deeper molecular response

By analogy with cytogenetic response assessment, the term complete molecular response (CMR) is frequently used to describe patients in whom there is no detectable *BCR–ABL* by RQ-PCR. As CMR is dependent on the detection limit of RQ-PCR, we prefer the term 'undetectable minimal residual disease' (UMRD). On imatinib the proportion of patients with UMRD increases progressively over time, and may be as high as 50% after 5 years [35]. This group of patients has attracted considerable interest since prospective multicenter studies have shown that around 40% of patients with UMRD for at least 2 years were able to stop imatinib and remain in treatment-free remission [36,37]. Similar studies are being conducted in patients treated with nilotinib and dasatinib.

The lower limit of detection of the RQ-PCR assay (commonly termed "sensitivity") varies between laboratories, and even between samples processed in the same batch on the same day in a single laboratory. This variability reflects pre-analytical variables including variation in white cell count, sample degradation (especially important where samples are transported long distances to a central laboratory), and analytical variables, such as enzyme activity and assay design [18,20,21,38].

There is a need for definitions of deep molecular response that are unambiguous and reproducible. Cross and colleagues proposed consensus guidelines for the reporting of samples with low level MRD or UMRD. MR4.0, for example, is used to describe a patient with UMRD with a limit of detection of at least four-log or detectable BCR–ABL at a level that is equal to or less than 0.01% [39]. The first prospective imatinib cessation studies required undetectable BCR–ABL and at least MR4.5 (BCR–ABL ≤0.0032%) as an inclusion criterion. Several subsequent clinical trials of treatment-free remission have adopted MR4.5 (without the need for UMRD) as a slightly less stringent, but more reproducible entry criterion. Less stringent criteria have been proposed for use in the ENESTFreedom and DASFREE trials [40,41].

Rising *BCR–ABL* levels

Most studies of TKI resistance have reported fold increases in BCR–ABL levels as evidence of loss of response. The extent of change that is significant varies between laboratories, and also varies with the BCR–ABL level, due to higher imprecision at lower levels of MRD. At BCR–ABL levels of >0.1% even an experienced laboratory will consider changes of up to twofold to be within the confidence limits of the test, and in some laboratories this range may be up to 10-fold. At lower levels of disease (below the level of MMR) the imprecision will be greater due to stochastic effects near the limit of detection. Each laboratory should determine the imprecision of its assay, and the clinicians who use that assay should be aware of what constitutes a clinically meaningful change. A significant increase in BCR–ABL should trigger a review of treatment compliance and/or a screen for kinase domain mutations.

The fold rise alone can be misleading if the interval between tests is variable. For example, an increase from 1% to 10% in one month would be more concerning than the same increase occurring over 6 months.

The doubling time is calculated using the fold change and the interval between tests. In chronic phase CML the doubling time of *BCR–ABL* when TKI treatment is stopped is around 10–14 days [42,43]. Similar doubling times are observed in patients developing blast crisis. Thus, a short doubling time raises the suspicion of poor drug adherence if blastic transformation has been excluded. Longer doubling times are characteristic of emerging drug resistance due to kinase domain mutations, but could also be an indicator of poor compliance with the doubling time inversely proportional to the number of missed doses [44].

Indications for mutation testing

The development of point mutations in the kinase domain of *BCR–ABL* is the most commonly identified cause of resistance to therapy with *ABL* kinase inhibitors [45–48]. Around half of patients in whom resistance occurs after an initial response (secondary resistance) are found to harbor kinase domain mutations. By contrast, direct sequencing of the kinase domain in newly diagnosed chronic phase CML patients never identifies mutations, although polymorphisms can sometimes cause confusion. Mutations arise more commonly in patients commencing imatinib in the late chronic phase and in the accelerated phase. Mutations are extremely rare in patients with primary resistance to imatinib, and alternative mechanisms of resistance (such as amplification of the Ph chromosome) must be involved. Once primary resistance is established there is a higher risk of point mutations developing in the kinase domain to further impair response to TKI therapy.

Screening for mutations is recommended in patients with a poor response to TKIs (eg, *BCR–ABL* >10% after 3 months of treatment), and in patients with secondary resistance. The incidence of mutations in patients with a greater than twofold rise in *BCR–ABL* (above the level of MMR) was approximately 60% in a series of patients tested in our laboratory [49]. By contrast, <1% of patients with stable or falling *BCR–ABL* levels had a detectable mutation. The degree of increase in *BCR–ABL* that should trigger mutation screening will vary between laboratories, as discussed above [49].

The presence of multiple mutations in CML may carry an especially adverse prognosis. This is particularly so when compound mutations are present within a single clone – as opposed to a mixture of clones, each carrying a single mutation. Compound mutations may still result in TKI resistance even with more potent drugs, such as ponatinib [50]. Sanger sequencing cannot reliably distinguish between compound mutations and multiple clones with a mixture of individual mutations. Massively parallel sequencing of the *ABL* kinase domain can identify mutations in cis, and may have a role in kinase domain mutation screening [51].

Pharmacokinetics

The measurement of imatinib drug levels in the plasma of CML patients has some clinical utility. Patients with lower drug levels (<1000 ng/mL) are less likely to achieve MMR [52]. Drug levels may be useful to investigate suspected non-compliance or therapeutic drug interactions – for example, if a new drug induces the hepatic clearance of imatinib. Data on the therapeutic drug monitoring of newer TKIs remain scarce.

Monitoring protocol in different clinical settings

Tyrosine kinase inhibitor treatment of chronic phase chronic myeloid leukemia

Blood counts should be monitored every 1–2 weeks until CHR is achieved because some patients will develop severe cytopenia requiring transfusion or granulocyte-colony stimulating factor (G-CSF) support. This is not due to a classical myelosuppressive effect of the TKI, but reflects delayed recovery of normal hematopoiesis following clearance of the leukemic cells. The development of significant cytopenia after CHR is uncommon and blood counts may be required only every 3 months for chronic phase patients on continuing therapy.

Cytogenetic analysis may be useful to confirm CCyR, typically after 6 months. This is especially important where *BCR–ABL* levels remain above the threshold of 1% after 6 months of therapy. Once MMR is achieved there is no indication for further marrow studies unless molecular response is lost or cytopenia develops and warrants investigation. As a minimum we recommend bone marrow examination as a baseline assessment for all patients; and testing every 3 months for patients with ≥10% *BCR–ABL*, as this group has the highest risk of disease progression.

Molecular monitoring is typically performed every 3 months. Monitoring should be performed more frequently in specific situations: for example poor response, suspected noncompliance, or introduction of concomitant medications that might interfere with the availability of the TKI. The doubling time of CML is such that with uncontrolled disease a one-log rise in *BCR–ABL* would occur in one month.

Tyrosine kinase inhibitor treatment of accelerated phase and blast crisis chronic myeloid leukemia

It is fortunate that advanced phase CML is now rather uncommon, but this means that there are limited data on which to base management recommendations. In accelerated phase and blast crisis CML the risk of TKI resistance is considerably higher than in chronic phase CML, and therefore more frequent monitoring may be warranted. In the accelerated phase bone marrow examination (with cytogenetic analysis) should be performed every 3 months. Molecular monitoring at shorter intervals – every 4–6 weeks – may be warranted until *BCR–ABL* levels fall to <10%. Due to the higher rate of clonal evolution a significant increase in *BCR–ABL* should trigger cytogenetic evaluation of the bone marrow as well as screening for kinase domain mutations, which are more frequent in advanced phase disease.

In blast crisis CML, where blasts may localize preferentially to the marrow, *BCR–ABL* levels may be lower in the blood than in the marrow. Patients in blast crisis with no detectable *BCR–ABL* in the peripheral blood should have RQ-PCR performed on the bone marrow aspirate for confirmation. This is in contrast to chronic phase CML where bone marrow RQ-PCR offers no additional sensitivity, and is not recommended [37]. In very rare cases chloroma (extramedullary leukemia) can occur despite stable *BCR–ABL* levels in the blood.

Allogeneic stem cell transplantation

Most patients allografted for chronic phase CML will have UMRD by 6 months post-transplant. Patients who still have detectable *BCR–ABL* after this time have a higher risk of relapse [53]. RQ-PCR monitoring is recommended every 3 months until stable UMRD is confirmed. For patients with this level of response the risk of relapse is so low that monitoring every 6 months or less may be sufficient. Very late relapses post-allograft have been reported, so some level of ongoing monitoring is required to enable timely intervention.

References

1   O'Brien SG, Guilhot F, Larson RA, et al. Imatinib compared with interferon and low-dose cytarabine for newly diagnosed chronic-phase chronic myeloid leukemia. *N Engl J Med*. 2003;348:994-1004.

2   Guilhot F, Chastang C, Michallet M, et al. Interferon alfa-2b combined with cytarabine versus interferon alone in chronic myelogenous leukemia. French Chronic Myeloid Leukemia Study Group. *N Engl J Med*. 1997;337:223-229.

3   Rosti G, Testoni N, Martinelli G, Baccarani M. The cytogenetic response as a surrogate marker of survival. *Semin Hematol*. 2003;40:56-61.

4   Anastasi J, Feng J, Le Beau MM, Larson RA, Rowley JD, Vardiman JW. The relationship between secondary chromosomal abnormalities and blast transformation in chronic myelogenous leukemia. *Leukemia*. 1995;9:628-633.

5   Kantarjian HM, Smith TL, McCredie KB, et al. Chronic myelogenous leukemia: a multivariate analysis of the associations of patient characteristics and therapy with survival. *Blood*. 1985;66:1326-1335.

6   Kantarjian HM, Dixon D, Keating MJ, et al. Characteristics of accelerated disease in chronic myelogenous leukemia. *Cancer*. 1988;61:1441-1446.

7   Marktel S, Marin D, Foot N, et al. Chronic myeloid leukemia in chronic phase responding to imatinib: the occurrence of additional cytogenetic abnormalities predicts disease progression. *Haematologica*. 2003;88:260-267.

8   O'Dwyer ME, Mauro MJ, Blasdel C, et al. Clonal evolution and lack of cytogenetic response are adverse prognostic factors for hematologic relapse of chronic phase CML patients treated with imatinib mesylate. *Blood*. 2004;103:451-455.

9   Bain BJ. Bone marrow biopsy morbidity and mortality: 2002 data. *Clin Lab Haematol*. 2004;26:315-318.

10   Eikelboom JW. Bone marrow biopsy in thrombocytopenic or anticoagulated patients. *Br J Haematol*. 2005;129:562-563.

11   Branford S, Hughes TP, Rudzki Z. Monitoring chronic myeloid leukaemia therapy by real-time quantitative PCR in blood is a reliable alternative to bone marrow cytogenetics. *Br J Haematol*. 1999;107:587-599.

12   Lange T, Bumm T, Otto S, et al. Quantitative reverse transcription polymerase chain reaction should not replace conventional cytogenetics for monitoring patients with chronic myeloid leukemia during early phase of imatinib therapy. *Haematologica*. 2004;89:49-57.

13   Cuneo A, Bigoni R, Emmanuel B, et al. Fluorescence in situ hybridization for the detection and monitoring of the Ph-positive clone in chronic myelogenous leukemia: comparison with metaphase banding analysis. *Leukemia*. 1998;12:1718-1723.

14   Kovitz C, Kantarjian H, Garcia-Manero G, Abruzzo LV, Cortes J. Myelodysplastic syndromes and acute leukemia developing after imatinib mesylate therapy for chronic myeloid leukemia. *Blood*. 2006;108:2811-2813.

15   Ross DM, Branford S, Moore S, Hughes TP. Limited clinical value of regular bone marrow cytogenetic analysis in imatinib-treated chronic phase CML patients monitored by RQ-PCR for BCR-ABL. *Leukemia*. 2006;20:664-670.

16   Ross DM, Jackson SR, Browett PJ. Philadelphia-negative secondary acute myeloid leukaemia during imatinib treatment for chronic phase chronic myeloid leukaemia. *Leuk Lymphoma*. 2007;48:1231-1233.

17   Terre C, Eclache V, Rousselot P, et al. Report of 34 patients with clonal chromosomal abnormalities in Philadelphia-negative cells during imatinib treatment of Philadelphia-positive chronic myeloid leukemia. *Leukemia*. 2004;18:1340-1346.

18   van der Velden VH, Boeckx N, Gonzalez M, et al. Differential stability of control gene and fusion gene transcripts over time may hamper accurate quantification of minimal residual disease--a study within the Europe Against Cancer Program. *Leukemia*. 2004;18:884-886.

19   Beillard E, Pallisgaard N, van der Velden VHJ, et al. Evaluation of candidate control genes for diagnosis and residual disease detection in leukemic patients using 'real-time' quantitative reverse-transcriptase polymerase chain reaction (RQ-PCR) - a Europe against cancer program. *Leukemia*. 2003;17:2474-2486.

20   Gabert J, Beillard E, van der Velden VHJ, et al. Standardization and quality control studies of 'real-time' quantitative reverse transcriptase polymerase chain reaction of fusion gene transcripts for residual disease detection in leukemia - a Europe Against Cancer program. *Leukemia*. 2003;17:2318-2357.

21   Branford S, Cross NC, Hochhaus A, et al. Rationale for the recommendations for harmonizing current methodology for detecting *BCR-ABL* transcripts in patients with chronic myeloid leukaemia. *Leukemia*. 2006;20:1925-1930.

22   Hughes TP, Kaeda J, Branford S, et al. Frequency of major molecular responses to imatinib or interferon alfa plus cytarabine in newly diagnosed chronic myeloid leukemia. *N Engl J Med*. 2003;349:1423-1432.

23   Hughes T, Deininger M, Hochhaus A, et al. Monitoring CML patients responding to treatment with tyrosine kinase inhibitors: review and recommendations for harmonizing current methodology for detecting BCR-ABL transcripts and kinase domain mutations and for expressing results. *Blood*. 2006;108:28-37.

24   Branford S, Fletcher L, Cross NCP, et al. Validation of the international scale for measurement of BCR-ABL by RQ-PCR based on deriving laboratory-specific conversion factors. *Blood*. 2007;110.

25   White HE, Hedges J, Bendit I, et al. Establishment and validation of analytical reference panels for the standardization of quantitative BCR-ABL1 measurements on the international scale. *Clin Chem*. 2013;59:938-948.

26   Jobbagy Z, van Atta R, Murphy KM, Eshleman JR, Gocke CD. Evaluation of the Cepheid GeneXpert *BCR-ABL* assay. *J Mol Diagn*. 2007;9:220-227.

27   O'Brien S, Abboud CN, Akhtari M, et al. NCC Clinical Practice Guidelines in Oncology: Chronic myelogenous leukemia, version 4. 2013. http://www.nccn.org/clinical.asp. Accessed April 8, 2014.

28   Wang L, Pearson K, Pillitteri L, Ferguson JE, Clark RE. Serial monitoring of BCR-ABL by peripheral blood real-time polymerase chain reaction predicts the marrow cytogenetic response to imatinib mesylate in chronic myeloid leukaemia. *Br J Haematol*. 2002;118:771-777.

29   Merx K, Muller MC, Kreil S, et al. Early reduction of BCR-ABL mRNA transcript levels predicts cytogenetic response in chronic phase CML patients treated with imatinib after failure of interferon alpha. *Leukemia*. 2002;16:1579-1583.

30   Hughes TP, Hochhaus A, Branford S. Long-term prognostic significance of early molecular response to imatinib in newly diagnosed chronic myeloid leukemia: an analysis from the International Randomized Study of Interferon and STI571 (IRIS). *Blood*. 2010;116:3758-3765.

31   Hanfstein B, Muller MC, Hehlmann R, et al. Early molecular and cytogenetic response is predictive for long-term progression-free and overall survival in chronic myeloid leukemia (CML). *Leukemia*. 2012;26:2096-2102.

32   Marin D, Ibrahim AR, Lucas C, et al. Assessment of *BCR-ABL*1 transcript levels at 3 months is the only requirement for predicting outcome for patients with chronic myeloid leukemia treated with tyrosine kinase inhibitors. *J Clin Oncol*. 2012;30:232-238.

33   Branford S, Yeung DT, Parker WT, et al. Prognosis for patients with CML and >10% BCR-ABL1 after 3 months of imatinib depends on the rate of BCR-ABL1 decline. *Blood*. 2014;124: 511-518

34   Hanfstein B, Shlyakhto V, Lauseker M, et al. Velocity of early BCR-ABL transcript elimination as an optimized predictor of outcome in chronic myeloid leukemia (CML) patients in chronic phase on treatment with imatinib. *Leukemia*. 2014; doi:10.1038/leu.2014.153 [Epub ahead of print].

35   Branford S, Seymour J, Grigg A, et al. BCR-ABL messenger RNA levels continue to decline in patients with chronic phase chronic myeloid leukemia treated with imatinib for more than 5 years and approximately half of all first-line treated patients have stable undetectable BCR-ABL using strict sensitivity criteria. *Clinical Cancer Research*. 2007;13:7080.

36   Mahon FX, Rea D, Guilhot J, et al. Discontinuation of imatinib in patients with chronic myeloid leukaemia who have maintained complete molecular remission for at least 2 years: the prospective, multicentre Stop Imatinib (STIM) trial. *Lancet Oncol*. 2010;11:1029-1035.

37   Ross DM, Branford S, Seymour JF, et al. Safety and efficacy of imatinib cessation for CML patients with stable undetectable minimal residual disease: results from the TWISTER study. *Blood*. 2013;122:515-522.

38   Thorn I, Olsson-Stromberg U, Ohlsen C, et al. The impact of RNA stabilization on minimal residual disease assessment in chronic myeloid leukemia. *Haematologica*. 2005;90:1471-1476.

39   Cross NC, White HE, Muller MC, Saglio G, Hochhaus A. Standardized definitions of molecular response in chronic myeloid leukemia. *Leukemia*. 2012;26:2172-2175.

40   Niliotinib Treatment-free Remission Study in CML (Chronic Myeloid Leukemia) Patients ENESTFreedom. http://clinicaltrials.gov/ct2/show/NCT01784068?term=ENESTfreedom&rank=1. Accessed 26 June 2014.

41   Open-Label Study Evaluating Dasatinib Therapy Discontinuation in Patients With Chronic Phase Chronic Myeloid Leukemia With Stable Complete Molecular Response (DASFREE). http://clinicaltrials.gov/ct2/show/NCT01850004?term=DASFREE&rank=1. Accessed 26 June 2014.

42   Michor F, Hughes TP, Iwasa Y, et al. Dynamics of chronic myeloid leukaemia. *Nature*. 2005;435:1267-1270.

43   Roeder I, Horn M, Glauche I, Hochhaus A, Mueller MC, Loeffler M. Dynamic modeling of imatinib-treated chronic myeloid leukemia: functional insights and clinical implications. *Nat Med*. 2006;12:1181-1184.

44   Branford S, Yeung DT, Prime JA, et al. *BCR-ABL1* doubling times more reliably assess the dynamics of CML relapse compared with the *BCR-ABL1* fold rise: implications for monitoring and management. *Blood*. 2012;119:4264-4271.

45   Branford S, Rudzki Z, Walsh S, et al. High frequency of point mutations clustered within the adenosine triphosphate-binding region of BCR/ABL in patients with chronic myeloid leukemia or Ph-positive acute lymphoblastic leukemia who develop imatinib (STI571) resistance. *Blood*. 2002;99:3472-3475.

46   Shah NP, Nicoll JM, Nagar B, et al. Multiple *BCR-ABL* kinase domain mutations confer polyclonal resistance to the tyrosine kinase inhibitor imatinib (STI571) in chronic phase and blast crisis chronic myeloid leukemia. *Cancer Cell*. 2002;2:117-125.

47   Gorre ME, Mohammed M, Ellwood K, et al. Clinical resistance to STI-571 cancer therapy caused by BCR-ABL gene mutation or amplification. *Science*. 2001;293:876-880.

48   Al-Ali HK, Heinrich MC, Lange T, et al. High incidence of BCR-ABL kinase domain mutations and absence of mutations of the PDGFR and KIT activation loops in CML patients with secondary resistance to imatinib. *Hematol J*. 2004;5:55-60.

49   Branford S, Rudzki Z, Parkinson I, et al. Real-time quantitative PCR analysis can be used as a primary screen to identify patients with CML treated with imatinib who have BCR-ABL kinase domain mutations. *Blood*. 2004;104:2926-2932.

50 O'Hare T, Shakespeare WC, Zhu X, et al. AP24534, a pan-BCR-ABL inhibitor for chronic myeloid leukemia, potently inhibits the T315I mutant and overcomes mutation-based resistance. *Cancer Cell*. 2009;16:401-412.

51 Soverini S, De Benedittis C, Machova Polakova K, et al. Unraveling the complexity of tyrosine kinase inhibitor-resistant populations by ultra-deep sequencing of the *BCR–ABL* kinase domain. *Blood*. 2013;122:1634-1648.

52 Picard S, Titier K, Etienne G, et al. Trough imatinib plasma levels are associated with both cytogenetic and molecular responses to standard-dose imatinib in chronic myeloid leukemia. *Blood*. 2007;109:3496-3499.

53 Radich JP, Gehly G, Gooley T, et al. Polymerase chain reaction detection of the BCR-ABL fusion transcript after allogeneic marrow transplantation for chronic myeloid leukemia: results and implications in 346 patients. *Blood*. 1995;85:2632-2638.

Chapter 4

Management of patients with chronic myeloid leukemia

Current approach to treatment

As recently as the 1990s the approach to chronic myeloid leukemia (CML) treatment was to allograft those who were eligible and palliate those who were not. Palliation with alpha interferon (IFNα) could prolong survival substantially for the 15–30% of patients who had IFNα-responsive disease but quality of life for these patients was often markedly impaired. Overall, the selective use of IFNα shifted the median survival from about 4 years to 5 years [1]. However, the trajectory for most patients was still a gradual decline towards accelerated disease and eventual blast crisis. Today, the expectation for newly diagnosed CML patients is that tyrosine kinase inhibitor (TKI) therapy will achieve long-term (perhaps indefinite) disease control in most patients, and that eventually some patients may even maintain remission without ongoing TKI therapy. The goals have shifted dramatically, which makes the early management of CML patients much more crucial than it used to be. The consequences of poor management may be a lost opportunity for a CML patient to live a long and fully active life. However, even with the best management some patients (5–10%) will progress early to blast crisis, some will fail to achieve an adequate response or lose response to frontline TKI therapy (15–20%), and a few of these will be refractory to all TKI therapy (around 5–10%). There is a danger that clinicians with limited experience and understanding of CML biology and therapy will manage

© Springer International Publishing Switzerland 2014
T.P. Hughes et al., *Handbook of Chronic Myeloid Leukemia*,
DOI 10.1007/978-3-319-08350-6_4

drug-related toxicities poorly, leading to frequent interruptions and inappropriate long-term use of suboptimal TKI doses. Poor drug adherence, in some cases related to inadequate education and motivation of the patient, can also lead to inadequate exposure to TKI therapy in the crucial first year of therapy. Inconsistent molecular monitoring, or the use of molecular laboratories with poor quality control, can compound these problems by leading to delayed action in response to emerging or actual TKI failure. Overall, outcomes for CML patients can be markedly inferior in these circumstances.

Which tyrosine kinase inhibitor to use?

After confirming the diagnosis of chronic phase CML the first step is to decide on the best TKI therapy for that patient. In many countries the TKIs imatinib, nilotinib and dasatinib are locally approved for frontline therapy and the clinician may have a choice of all three drugs. While it would be tempting to use the TKI that is most familiar to the clinician it is probably not optimal management to select the same drug in every case. There is emerging evidence that in specific circumstances one TKI may be a better choice for a particular patient. Detailed knowledge of the efficacy and safety profile of each TKI, the susceptibility of the patient to toxicities, and clarity about the therapeutic goals should all be weighed carefully when choosing the frontline TKI. Here, we review the strengths and weaknesses of the three currently available frontline TKIs.

Imatinib

The first TKI that was clinically developed for a human cancer, imatinib, is an effective and remarkably safe option for many CML patients. Treatment with imatinib results in a stable major molecular response (MMR) in around 60% of patients with CML, is poorly tolerated in around 20%, and a further 20% of patients do not achieve or maintain an optimal response [2]. A disadvantage of imatinib is that it is significantly less potent at inhibiting *BCR–ABL* than nilotinib or dasatinib. Data from in vitro studies as well as clinical observations have shown that inadequate kinase inhibition in patients receiving imatinib is not uncommon, and is associated with inferior response [3,4]. This might be because of a failure in achieving adequate blood levels of imatinib: plasma trough drug levels below 1000 ng/mL are associated with an inferior response [5,6]. However, this is not the only contributing factor to suboptimal imatinib-induced kinase inhibition in leukemia. Inadequate cellular uptake of drugs, even in the presence of adequate drug levels, may arise because of reduced activity of the organic cation transporter 1 (OCT-1) influx pump [7]. Low activity of OCT-1 is observed in the majority of patients who fail to achieve optimal response to imatinib [7–10]. Another disadvantage of imatinib as a frontline drug in chronic phase CML, compared with the more potent newer TKIs, is susceptibility to a great range of kinase domain mutations (see Chapter 5) that commonly lead to imatinib resistance [11]. Around 5–10% of CML patients on frontline imatinib therapy develop kinase domain mutations that are usually associated with a loss of response. Patients who receive imatinib experience some degree of impairment in quality of life: common problems are excessive fluid retention, muscle cramps, or gastrointestinal disturbance including nausea and diarrhea.

However, there are potential advantages to using imatinib frontline. Unlike nilotinib and dasatinib, there have been few significant organ toxicities reported after long-term exposure to imatinib. The other important advantage, especially in locations in which drug costs are a crucial consideration, is the availability of generic imatinib in many countries either now or over the next few years.

The International Randomized Study of Interferon and STI571 (IRIS) trial showed an 8-year survival for imatinib recipients of 85%; however survival was 93% if only CML-related deaths were considered. For the 55% of patients who remained on imatinib in the IRIS trial at 8 years, nearly all had achieved at least a complete cytogenetic response (CCyR), and the progression rate after the first 3 years of therapy was close to zero [2,12]. So far, no other TKI that has been used as frontline therapy has demonstrated superior survival compared with imatinib.

There is no evidence from randomized studies that a dose of imatinib higher than 400 mg results in superior efficacy. Randomized studies [13,14] comparing 400 mg with 800 mg per day did not demonstrate a clear advantage with the higher dose, except in the case of the German CML IV study [15] in which higher rates of molecular response were achieved in patients randomized to 800 mg/day compared with patients given 400 mg/day. However, no significant improvement in progression free or overall survival has been observed in any of the randomized trials comparing higher dose with standard dose imatinib, including the German CML IV study.

Nilotinib

Nilotinib is structurally similar to imatinib although its affinity for *BCR–ABL* and off-target effects are different. Nilotinib binds to the kinase domain of *BCR–ABL*, with greater affinity than imatinib and is less vulnerable to kinase domain mutations. Only five mutations are of major concern in the context of nilotinib treatment (*T315I, F359V, E255K, E255V,* and *Y253H*); these mutations emerge most frequently on frontline or second-line nilotinib therapy, and their presence is a contraindication to the use of nilotinib after failure of another TKI [16,17].

In the Evaluating Nilotinib Efficacy and Safety in Clinical Trials – Newly Diagnosed Patients (ENESTnd) study both nilotinib arms (300 mg and 400 mg twice daily [BID]) demonstrated a higher rate of cytogenetic and molecular response and a lower rate of progression compared with imatinib 400 mg daily [16]. After follow-up of 4 years, MMR and $MR^{4.5}$ rates were higher in both the nilotinib arms compared with the imatinib arm. Estimated 4-year rates of freedom from progression to accelerated phase/blast crisis in the study (including events during follow-up after discontinuation) were 97% (p=0.05) and 98% (p=0.0074) in the 300 mg and 400 BID nilotinib arms, respectively, compared with 93% on the imatinib arm. However, after 4 years the lower risk of transformation has not translated into a survival advantage when all patients are considered [18,19]. The day to day toxicity of nilotinib is generally mild – edema is rare and gastrointestinal toxicity is uncommon. Elevated lipase and abnormal liver function tests are each observed in 5–10% of patients but do not often lead to discontinuation of therapy. A significant concern related to the use of nilotinib is the occurrence of vascular events, including peripheral arterial occlusive disease, coronary artery disease, and cerebrovascular disease, as well as hyperglycemia and hypercholesterolemia. Case reports of serious progressive vascular events emerged first, but most of these patients had multiple risk factors for vascular disease [20,21]. We now have evidence from the ENESTnd study [22] that the incidence of these three types of vascular events appears to be higher on both nilotinib arms than the imatinib arm (Table 4.1).

Events were seen most commonly in patients with a history of previous vascular events or diabetes. The significance of this problem with long-term exposure to nilotinib remains to be determined but it is certainly an issue to keep in mind when selecting a TKI for a patient with risk factors for atherosclerotic disease. If nilotinib is chosen as frontline therapy then careful attention to cardiovascular risk factors is warranted. Nilotinib is clearly associated with hyperglycemia, possibly by inducing insulin resistance. In the ENESTnd trial 20% of patients on the nilotinib 300 mg BID arm who were not diabetic at baseline were diabetic by 3 years, compared with 9% on the imatinib arm [23]. Diabetic and pre-diabetic patients who are starting nilotinib therapy should be closely monitored. Elevations in total cholesterol and low-density lipoprotein (LDL) cholesterol have been well documented in patients treated with nilotinib and many become eligible for lipid lowering agents according to national cardiology guidelines.

Finally, it is important to note that any clinically significant vascular event occurring on nilotinib therapy should signal the urgent need to review the optimal choice of ongoing TKI therapy, and in most cases a switch to another TKI would be indicated.

Dasatinib

Dasatinib has similar in vivo potency to nilotinib but a relatively short half-life, suggesting it would be optimally administered in two or three daily doses. However, the randomized SRC/ABL Tyrosine Kinase Inhibition Activity: Research Trial of BMS-354825 (START-R) demonstrated that twice-daily dosing offered no advantage in terms of efficacy and greater toxicity compared with once-daily dosing [24]. The frontline randomized trial DASatinib versus Imatinib Study In treatment-Naive CML patients (DASISION) compared dasatinib 100 mg daily with imatinib 400 mg daily. In this trial, patients receiving dasatinib showed superior early molecular responses compared with those receiving imatinib and dasatinib

Patients with an event n (%)	Nilotinib 300 mg BID n = 282				Nilotinib 400 mg BID n = 281				Imatinib 400 mg QD n = 283			
	Total n (%)	Y1–3 n	Y4 n	Y5 n	Total n (%)	Y1–3 n	Y4 n	Y5 n	Total n (%)	Y1–3 n	Y4 n	Y5 n
Peripheral arterial occlusive disease	7 (3)	4	0	3	7 (3)	3	2	2	0	0	0	0
Ischemic heart disease	11 (4)	9	2	0	24 (9)	11	3	10	5 (2)	3	0	2
Ischemic cerebrovascular events	4 (1)	2	1	1	9 (3)	4	1	4	1 (<1)	1	0	0
Total (%)	8				15				<3			

Table 4.1 Selected cardiac and vascular events by five years in the ENESTnd study. BID, twice daily; QD, once daily. Reproduced with permission from © Nature Publishing Group, 2012. All rights reserved. Larson et al [26]. Reproduced with permission from © American Society of Hematology, 2013. All rights reserved. Saglio et al [27]. Reproduced with permission from © American Society of Clinical Oncology, 2014. All rights reserved. Larson et al [28].

was generally well tolerated. The rate of progression was lower on the dasatinib arm, but no survival advantage has emerged thus far [25].

Similar numbers of kinase domain mutations have emerged following administration of imatinib and dasatinib in the DASISION trial. A higher number of *T315I* mutations have been observed in this trial on the dasatinb arm, in contrast to the ENESTnd trial in which *T315I* was seen in a similar number of patients in nilotinib and imatinib arms. The reasons for this difference are not clear, but may relate to the limited number of mutations that are resistant to dasatinib (*T315A, T315I, V299L, F317L*, and *F317I*) [11].

Only 10% of patients have withdrawn from the dasatinib arm of the DASISION study because of any adverse events. The main safety concern with dasatinib use compared with other TKIs relates to pleural effusions – pleural effusions occurred in approximately 25% of dasatinib-treated patients in the DASISION study. These events were usually grade I–II but frequently led to the use of diuretics and steroids, and the need to interrupt and/or reduce the dasatinib dose. Even in the fourth year of dasatinib therapy, new reports of pleural effusions were received from 5% of dasatinib recipients suggesting that the risk of these events does not diminish over time [25]. The incidence of pleural effusions is strongly age-dependent with rare reports in patients under 30, whereas over 50% of patients older than 70 develop pleural effusions. Of more concern are rare reports of pulmonary arterial hypertension (PAH), which is a potentially life-threatening condition [29]. Nine cases were reported to the French PAH registry over a 4-year period. All but one of these cases improved markedly with dasatinib cessation; however none of these cases returned to normal pulmonary pressures. The incidence was estimated to be less than 1% in French patients receiving dasatinib [29]. Recent reports of echocardiogram results [30,31] on patients receiving dasatinib suggest that the rate of asymptomatic PAH may be higher than this but few patients have had angiographic confirmation of PAH. The extent of the problem with long-term exposure will need to be closely monitored.

Clonal lymphocytosis with large granular lymphocyte (LGL) morphology is not uncommon in dasatinib-treated patients, and has been associated with slightly superior response rates [32]. Whether this represents an anti-leukemic immune response induced by dasatinib, or non-specific immune dysregulation is unclear. Further work is needed to ascertain whether this phenomenon could be exploited to improve responses.

Summary

In summary, the choice at diagnosis is between imatinib, the first TKI to be approved for the treatment of CML, which is safe but only leads to long-term optimal response in about 60% of patients, and the more potent second-generation TKIs nilotinib and dasatinib that probably reduce the transformation risk but do not seem to offer a substantial benefit in terms of overall survival. Both nilotinib and dasatinib have some question marks regarding long-term toxicity, which should lead us to be cautious about their widespread frontline use without clear justification.

Determining the treatment goals

The long-term treatment goals for most patients with CML are: (1) a lifespan not shortened by CML or the therapy used to treat the CML; and (2) quality of life as close to normal as possible (Figure 4.1).

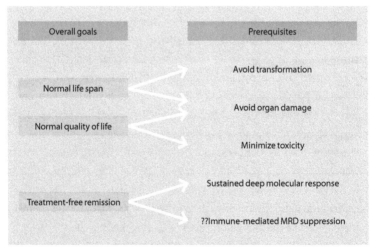

Figure 4.1 The goals and consequent prerequisites of frontline chronic myeloid leukemia therapy. When selecting frontline therapy for chronic myeloid leukemia three overall goals are generally accepted. These goals determine the five prerequisites for measuring whether those goals have been achieved. The TKIs that are available for frontline therapy can be assessed against these prerequisites. MRD, minimal residual disease; TKI, tyrosine kinase inhibitor.

To achieve the former goal the main prerequisites are avoidance of disease transformation and avoidance of major drug-induced organ toxicity. A normal quality of life requires avoidance of organ toxicity as well as minimizing the impact of TKI-related side effects. When comparing the three available frontline TKIs based on these criteria there is no clear advantage for one over the other (Figure 4.2).

However, for many patients today a third goal of therapy has emerged – that of treatment-free remission (TFR). The probable superiority of nilotinib and dasatinib in achieving TFR may be the strongest justification for using one of these two drugs as frontline therapy for some patients. While imatinib seems to be a safe drug over the course of 10–15 years of exposure, significant organ toxicities may be revealed with life-long exposure. Long-term exposure to nilotinib or dasatinib may be even more problematic. For women who wish to start a family the achievement of TFR is probably a particularly high priority because of the teratogenic potential of these agents.

Prerequisites	imatinib	nilotinib	dasatinib
Avoid transformation	5–8%	Lower	Lower
Avoid organ damage	Safe	Vascular events	PAH
Minimize toxcity	GI muscle	Rash pruritus	Pleural effusions
Sustained deep response	40%	Better	Better
??Immune control	40%	??	??

Figure 4.2 **Comparison between the three clinically available tyrosine kinase inhibitors in terms of their capacity to achieve the prerequisites of frontline therapy.** The advantage of the most potent TKIs, in terms of lower rates of transformation, needs to be considered alongside the added risk associated with these drugs with regards to possible organ toxicity. Improvement in the rates of deep molecular response will probably lead to higher rates of TFR with the more potent TKIs, which would provide a stronger justification for their frontline use. PAH, pulmonary arterial hypertension; TFR, treatment-free remission; TKI, tyrosine kinase inhibitor.

The evidence from the French Stop Imatinib (STIM) trial and the Australian TWISTER trial is fairly convincing – around 30–40% of CML patients who achieve a stable deep molecular response on imatinib can stop therapy and remain polymerase chain reaction (PCR)-negative for many years [33–35]. In fact, there have been only rare cases of late molecular recurrence in patients who remained PCR-negative in the long-term after imatinib cessation. Several hundred patients with CML have entered cessation studies and, to date, no reports of drug resistance have emerged. Caution is warranted when considering TFR as a goal for younger patients because only a small minority of patients who receive frontline imatinib may ever achieve it. In an Australian study of over 400 patients with CML approximately 35% eventually achieved stable undetectable minimal residual disease (MRD) (previously called stable complete molecular response [CMR]; denotes the absence of *BCR–ABL* by RQ-PCR after 2 years of monitoring with sensitivity of at least 4.5 logs as determined by the number of control gene transcripts amplified) [36]. Of these patients around 30–40% are likely to remain in stable molecular remission in the long term if imatinib therapy is ceased. Therefore, in a population of patients with CML who receive frontline imatinib it is probable that less than 15% will eventually achieve TFR. An important question is whether a substantially higher rate of TFR will be achieved if the more potent TKIs are used as frontline or second-line therapy. The potential to improve the rate of TFR may be the strongest argument in favor of using nilotinib or dasatinib as frontline therapy in younger patients regardless of risk profile.

A French study that assessed the molecular disease recurrence rate in patients ceasing second-generation TKI therapy after achieving stable deep molecular responses showed encouraging results. Patients who switched to nilotinib or dasatinib because of intolerance to imatinib and who then achieved stable CMR had a 60% probability of remaining in MMR following treatment cessation [37]. Given that the achievement of deep molecular response seems to be higher with second-generation TKIs than with imatinib, then the overall rate of TFR achieved by using frontline nilotinib or dasatinib may therefore be significantly higher than the rate observed following imatinib treatment (Table 4.2). Based on these data, second-generation drugs used as frontline therapy might achieve a higher rate of TFR overall. However, mature data are needed before this can be definitively stated.

Achieving treatment goals

When considering frontline therapy in the older patient for whom TFR is not usually a major goal, imatinib remains the most suitable choice. The ENESTnd, DASISION and Eastern Cooperative Oncology Group (ECOG) studies [18,28,40] were all powered to identify a superior rate of cytogenetic or molecular response for the investigational TKI at 12 months. While all of these studies have shown superior response rates for the more potent TKIs compared with imatinib, none has demonstrated a survival advantage over imatinib in the frontline setting. If

TKI approach	CMR rate (%)	Successful cessation rate (%)	Overall achievement of TFR (%)
1. Imatinib*	40	30	12
2A: Imatinib-NIL/DAS conservative estimate†	60	20	12
2B: Imatinib-NIL/DAS best case estimate†	70	60	42
3A: NIL/DAS conservative estimate‡	60	20	12
3B: NIL/DAS best case estimate‡	80	60	48

*See references [33–35] for the actual rate.
†Estimates based on patients starting with imatinib and then switching over to nilotinib or dasatinib if they do not achieve a deep MR on imatinib. 2A is a conservative estimate of the rates based on the assumption that there are a fixed number of CML patients who will achieve treatment-free remission regardless of which TKI they receive. 2B is the best estimate based on extrapolating figures of stable undetectable minimal residual disease and stable remission after cessation in recently presented trials [33–37].
‡Estimates based on patients receiving nilotinib or dasatinib frontline. 3A is a conservative estimate of the rates based on the assumption that there are a fixed number of CML patients who will achieve treatment-free remission regardless of which TKI they receive. 3B is the best estimate based on extrapolating figures of stable undetectable minimal residual disease and stable remission after cessation in recently presented trials [15,33,38].

Table 4.2 Actual rates of stable undetectable minimal residue disease and sustained remission after cessation, and calculated rates of overall treatment-free remission for imatinib; estimated rates are for second-generation tyrosine kinase inhibitors. CML, chronic myeloid leukemia; CMR, complete molecular response; DAS, dasatinib; NIL, nilotinib; TFR, treatment-free remission; TKI, tyrosine kinase inhibitor; UMRD, undetectable minimal residue disease. Reproduced with permission from © American Society of Hematology, 2013. All rights reserved. Hughes, White [39].

imatinib is the frontline choice then it is still crucial that cytogenetic and molecular response is closely monitored. Under the revised European LeukemiaNet (ELN) recommendations [41], criteria for failure represent an indication to switch therapy because survival is likely to be inferior if therapy is maintained (Table 4.3). The molecular targets in this circumstance should be *BCR–ABL* values of <10% by 6 months and <1% by 12 months. A *BCR–ABL* level <0.1% (MMR) by 18 months is also optimal; however the additional benefit of achieving MMR by 18 months, compared with achieving CCyR or its molecular equivalent, <1% *BCR–ABL* International Scale (IS), with regard to the long-term prospects of survival is only small. There is a 1% versus 3% risk of death over the subsequent 5 years for patients who, at 18 months, achieved *BCR–ABL* levels of <0.1%, and those patients whose *BCR–ABL* values are between 1% and 0.1%, respectively [42].

Identifying high-risk patients based on early molecular response

The strategy behind the Therapeutic Intensification in De Novo Leukemia II (TIDEL II) study in Australia and New Zealand was to maximize the use of imatinib and only use more potent TKIs (in this study, nilotinib) when

	Optimal	Warning	Failure
Baseline	NA	High risk or CCA/Ph+, major route	NA
3 months	*BCR–ABL*1 ≤10% and/or Ph+ ≤35%	*BCR–ABL*1 >10% and/or Ph+ 36–95%	Non-CHR and/or Ph+ >95%
6 months	*BCR–ABL* 1 <1% and/or Ph+ 0	*BCR–ABL* 1 1–10% and/or Ph+ 1–35%	*BCR–ABL* 1 >10% and/or Ph+ >35%
12 months	*BCR–ABL* 1 ≤0%	*BCR–ABL* 1 >0.1–1%	*BCR–ABL* 1 >1% and/or Ph+ >0
Then, and at any time	*BCR–ABL* 1 ≤0.1%	CCA/Ph– (–7 or 7q–)	Loss of CHR Loss of CCyR Confirmed loss of MMR Mutations CCA/Ph+

Table 4.3 European LeukemiaNet recommendations for defining response to frontline tyrosine kinase inhibitor therapy. *BCR–ABL*, breakpoint cluster region–Abelson oncogene; CCA, clonal chromosome abnormalities; CCyR, complete cytogenetic response; CHR, complete hematological response; MMR, major molecular response; NA, non-applicable. Reproduced with permission from © American Society of Hematology, 2013. All rights reserved. Baccarani et al [41].

there was evidence of imatinib intolerance or a high risk of progression. Frontline imatinib at a dose of 600 mg/day was given to all patients, and the molecular response at 3, 6, and 12 months was used to identify the high-risk patients, who were switched to nilotinib. Patients with >10% *BCR–ABL* at 3 months, >1% at 6 months, or >0.1% at 12 months were dose escalated to imatinib 800 mg. Patients who still failed to meet their molecular target 3 months later were switched to nilotinib (Cohort 1) or switched straight away to nilotinib (Cohort 2) if they did not achieve these targets [38]. Despite the early intensification of therapy applied in the TIDEL II study this approach does not rescue all patients from an adverse outcome. The rate of transformation for patients with >10% *BCR–ABL* at 3 months was over 10% and progression events amongst these high-risk patients were usually observed in the first 12 months. It is not known whether these patients would have achieved better outcomes if they had started frontline nilotinib therapy. In the ENESTnd study, adverse outcomes were observed for patients with >10% *BCR–ABL* at 3 months regardless of whether they received frontline nilotinib or imatinib. The risk of transformation was over 10% in all three arms and half of the progression events occurred prior to 6 months [38,43]. Overall, these observations suggest that the 3-month molecular response is a good indicator of the long-term probability of achieving a deep molecular response and the short-term risk of progression, but has limited utility as an identifier of high-risk patients who may benefit from intensifying therapy, possibly because by 3 months it is too late to reverse the pathway to early transformation.

Risk-adapted therapy

It is also important to consider the prognostic score of the individual when choosing frontline therapy. There are three scoring systems that are currently applied in CML – Sokal, Hasford, and European Treatment and Outcome Study for CML (EUTOS), and there is no clear indication that one is superior to the others [41]. For all three scoring systems, a high score is associated with a higher risk of progression to accelerated phase or to blast crisis. As both nilotinib and dasatinib have been shown to reduce the risk of CML progression these drugs might be preferred over imatinib in this group of high-risk patients. Figure 4.3 demonstrates a schema that sets out how to decide which frontline therapy would be optimal.

Other predictive markers have been investigated and may prove to be superior to the current risk scores or, more likely, may provide additional predictive value, but these require further validation.

Other promising frontline approaches
Combination pegylated interferon plus a tyrosine kinase inhibitor

IFN was the best drug available for CML prior to the TKI era. While monotherapy with IFN is rarely indicated in any circumstance except pregnancy, there is renewed interest in using pegylated IFN in combination with a TKI. The German CML IV study [44] did not demonstrate an advantage for patients who were given imatinib plus (non-pegylated) IFN; however two other randomized studies showed significantly better responses in patients given pegylated IFN with imatinib. Both the French Prospective International Randomised Trial (SPIRIT) and the Nordic

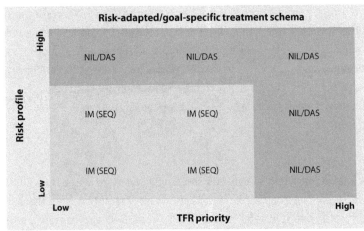

Figure 4.3 Risk-adapted and goal-specific treatment schema for individualizing the frontline therapy for a chronic myeloid leukemia patient. This proposed schema assesses the priority of a patient for achieving TFR as well as their biological risk profile (eg, Sokal score). Using this risk-adapted and goal-specific schema, patients confirmed as either a high risk or a high priority to achieve TFR would receive a second-generation TKI as frontline therapy. CML, chronic myeloid leukemia; DAS, dasatinib; IM, imatinib; NIL, nilotinib; SEQ, sequence; TFR, treatment-free remission; TKI, tyrosine kinase inhibitor.

studies [45] showed that relatively low doses of pegylated IFN given for several months in the first year were associated with superior rates of deep molecular response. No reduction in the probability of progression or death has been observed to date. This remains an experimental approach but may be a promising strategy to achieve deeper molecular responses and potentially recruit more patients to cessation studies, since the achievement of a deep molecular response is the main prerequisite for a trial of cessation.

References

1   Helhmann R, Berger U, Pfirrman M, et al. Randomized comparison of interferon alpha and hydroxyurea with hydroxyurea monotherapy in chronic myeloid leukemia (CML-study II): prolongation of survival by the combination of interferon alpha and hydroxyurea. *Leukemia*. 2003;17:1529-1537.

2   Hochhaus A, O'Brien SG, Guilhot F, et al. Six-year follow-up of patients receiving imatinib for the first-line treatment of chronic myeloid leukemia. *Leukemia*. 2009;23:1054-1061.

3   White D, Saunders V, Grigg A, et al. Measurement of in vivo BCR-ABL kinase inhibition to monitor imatinib-induced target blockade and predict response in chronic myeloid leukemia. *J Clin Oncol*. 2007;25:4445-4451.

4   White D, Saunders V, Lyons AB, et al. In vitro sensitivity to imatinib-induced inhibition of ABL kinase activity is predictive of molecular response in patients with de novo CML. *Blood*. 2005;106:2520-2526.

5   Larson RA, Druker BJ, Guilhot F, et al. Imatinib pharmacokinetics and its correlation with response and safety in chronic-phase chronic myeloid leukemia: a subanalysis of the IRIS study. *Blood*. 2008;111:4022-4028.

6   Picard S, Titier K, Etienne G, et al. Trough imatinib plasma levels are associated with both cytogenetic and molecular responses to standard-dose imatinib in chronic myeloid leukemia. *Blood*. 2007;109:3496-3499.

7   Thomas J, Wang L, Clark RE, Pirmohamed M. Active transport of imatinib into and out of cells: implications for drug resistance. *Blood*. 2004;104:3739-3745.

8   White DL, Saunders VA, Dang P, et al. OCT-1-mediated influx is a key determinant of the intracellular uptake of imatinib but not nilotinib (AMN107): reduced OCT-1 activity is the cause of low in vitro sensitivity to imatinib. *Blood*. 2006;108:697-704.

9   White DL, Radich J, Soverini S, et al. Chronic phase chronic myeloid leukemia patients with low OCT-1 activity randomized to high-dose imatinib achieve better responses and have lower failure rates than those randomized to standard-dose imatinib. *Haematologica*. 2012;97:907-914.

10   White DL, Saunders VA, Dang P, et al. Most CML patients who have a suboptimal response to imatinib have low OCT-1 activity: higher doses of imatinib may overcome the negative impact of low OCT-1 activity. *Blood*. 2007;110:4064-4072.

11   Branford S, Melo JV, Hughes TP. Selecting optimal second-line tyrosine kinase inhibitor therapy for chronic myeloid leukemia patients after imatinib failure: does the BCR-ABL mutation status really matter? *Blood*. 2009;114:5426-5435.

12   Deininger M, O'Brien SG, Guilhot F, et al. International Randomized Study of Interferon Vs STI571 (IRIS) 8-year follow up: sustained survival and low risk for progression or events in patients with newly diagnosed chronic myeloid leukemia in chronic phase (CML-CP) treated with imatinib. In: Proceedings from the 51st ASH Annual Meeting; December 5–8, 2009; New Orleans, LA. Abstract 1126.

13   Baccarani M, Rosti G, Castagnetti F, et al. Comparison of imatinib 400 mg and 800 mg daily in the front-line treatment of high-risk, Philadelphia-positive chronic myeloid leukemia: a European LeukemiaNet Study. *Blood*. 2009;113:4497-4504.

14   Cortes JE, Baccarani M, Guilhot F, et al. Phase III, randomized, open-label study of daily imatinib mesylate 400 mg versus 800 mg in patients with newly diagnosed, previously untreated chronic myeloid leukemia in chronic phase using molecular end points: tyrosine kinase inhibitor optimization and selectivity study. *J Clin Oncol*. 2010;28:424-430.

15   Hehlmann R, Lauseker M, Jung-Munkwitz S, et al. Tolerability-adapted imatinib 800 mg/d versus 400 mg/d versus 400 mg/d plus interferon-α in newly diagnosed chronic myeloid leukemia. *J Clin Oncol*. 2011;29:1634-1642.

16   Saglio G, Kim DW, Issaragrisil S, et al. Nilotinib versus imatinib for newly diagnosed chronic myeloid leukemia. *N Engl J Med*. 2010;362:2251-2259.

17   Hughes T, Saglio G, Branford S, et al. Impact of baseline BCR-ABL mutations on response to nilotinib in patients with chronic myeloid leukemia in chronic phase. *J Clin Oncol*. 2009;27:4204-4210.

18   Kantarjian HM, Hochhaus A, Saglio G, et al. Nilotinib versus imatinib for the treatment of patients with newly diagnosed chronic phase, Philadelphia chromosome-positive, chronic myeloid leukaemia: 24-month minimum follow-up of the phase 3 randomised ENESTnd trial. *Lancet Oncol*. 2011;12:841-851.

19   Larson R, Hochhaus A, Saglio G, et al. Nilotinib versus imatinib in patients (pts) with newly diagnosed chronic myeloid leukemia in chronic phase (CML-CP): ENESTnd 4-year (y) update. *J Clin Oncol*. 2013;31:suppl;abstr 7052.

20   Aichberger KJ, Herndlhofer S, Schernthaner GH, et al. Progressive peripheral arterial occlusive disease and other vascular events during nilotinib therapy in CML. *Am J Hematol*. 2011;86:533-539.

21   Kim TD, Rea D, Schwarz M, et al. Peripheral artery occlusive disease in chronic phase chronic myeloid leukemia patients treated with nilotinib or imatinib. *Leukemia*. 2013;27:1316-1321.

22   Hehlmann R, Lauseker M, Jung-Munkwitz J, et al. Tolerability-adapted imatinib 800 mg/d versus 400 mg/d versus 400 mg/d plus interferon-α in newly diagnosed chronic myeloid leukemia. *J Clin Oncol*. 2011;29:1634-1642.

23   Rea D, Gautier J-f, Breccia M, et al. Incidence of hyperglycemia by 3 years in patients (Pts) with newly diagnosed chronic myeloid leukemia in chronic phase (CML-CP) treated with nilotinib (NIL) or imatinib (IM) in ENESTnd [abstract]. *Blood (ASH Annual Meeting Abstracts)*. 2012;120:1686.

24   Kantarjian H, Pasquini R, Levy V, et al. Dasatinib or high-dose imatinib for chronic-phase chronic myeloid leukemia resistant to imatinib at a dose of 400 to 600 milligrams daily: two-year follow-up of a randomized phase 2 study (START-R). *Cancer*. 2009;115:4136-4147.

25   Kantarjian HM, Shah NP, Cortes JE, et al. Dasatinib or imatinib in newly diagnosed chronic-phase chronic myeloid leukemia: 2-year follow-up from a randomized phase 3 trial (DASISION). *Blood*. 2012;119:1123-1129.

26   Larson RA, Hochhaus A, Hughes TP, et al. Nilotinib vs imatinib in patients with newly diagnosed Philadelphia positive chronic myeloid leukemia in chronic phase: ENESTnd 3-year follow up. *Leukemia*. 2012;26:2197-2203.

27   Saglio G, Hochhaus A, Hughes TP, et al. ENESTnd update: Nilotinib (NIL) vs imatinib (IM) in patients (pts) with newly diagnosed chronic myeloid leukemia in chronic phase (CML-CP) and the impact of early molecular response (EMR) and Sokal risk at diagnosis on long-term outcomes. *Blood*. 2013;122:92.

28   Larson RA, Kim D-W, Jootar S, et al. ENESTnd 5-year (y) update: Long-term outcomes of patients (pts) with chronic myeloid leukemia in chronic phase (CML-CP) treated with frontline nilotinib (NIL) versus imatinib (IM). *J Clin Oncol (ASCO Annual Meeting Abstracts)*. 2014;32(suppl 15):7073.

29   Montani D, Bergot E, Günther S, et al. Pulmonary arterial hypertension in patients treated by dasatinib. *Circulation*. 2012;125:2128-2137.

30   Tatarczuch M, Seymour JF, Creati L, Januszewicz EH, Burbury K. Pulmonary hypertension
      (PHT) and pleural effusion during dasatinib therapy for CML frequently lead to drug
      withdrawal. *Blood*. 2013;122:1504.
31   Jeon Y-W, Lee S-E, Kim S-H, et al. Six-year follow-up of dasatinib-related pulmonary arterial
      hypertension (PAH) for chronic myeloid leukemia in single center. *Blood*. 2013;122:4017.
32   Matsuki E, Kumagai T, Inokuchi K, et al. Relative increase of lymphocytes as early as 1 month
      after initiation of dasatinib is a reliable predictor for achieving complete molecular response
      at 12 months in chronic phase CML patients treated with dasatinib [abstract]. *Blood (ASH
      Annual Meeting Abstracts)*. 2012;120:691.
33   Mahon FX, Rea D, Guilhot J, et al. Discontinuation of imatinib in patients with chronic
      myeloid leukaemia who have maintained complete molecular remission for at least 2 years:
      the prospective, multicentre Stop Imatinib (STIM) trial. *Lancet Oncol*. 2010;11:1029-1035.
34   Ross DM, Branford S, Seymour JF, et al. Patients with chronic myeloid leukemia who
      maintain a complete molecular response after stopping imatinib treatment have evidence
      of persistent leukemia by DNA PCR. *Leukemia*. 2010;24:1719-1724.
35   Ross DM, Branford S, Seymour JF, et al. Safety and efficacy of imatinib cessation for CML
      patients with stable undetectable minimal residual disease: results from the TWISTER Study.
      Blood. 2013;122:515-522.
36   Branford S, Yeung DT, Ross DM, et al. Early molecular response and female sex strongly
      predict stable undetectable BCR-ABL1, the criteria for imatinib discontinuation in patients
      with CML. *Blood*. 2013;121:3818-3824.
37   Rea D, Philippe Rousselot, Guilhot F, et al. Discontinuation of second generation (2G)
      tyrosine kinase inhibitors (TKI) in chronic phase (CP)-chronic myeloid leukemia (CML)
      patients with stable undetectable BCR-ABL transcripts[abstract]. *Blood (ASH Annual Meeting
      Abstracts)*. 2012;120:961.
38   Yeung DT, Osborn MP, White DL, et al. Early switch to nilotinib does not overcome the
      adverse outcome for CML patients failing to achieve early molecular response on imatinib,
      despite excellent overall outcomes in the TIDEL II trial[abstract]. *Blood (ASH Annual Meeting
      Abstracts)*. 2012;120:3771.
39   Hughes T, White D. Which TKI? An embarrassment of riches for chronic myeloid leukemia
      patients. *ASH Education Book*. 2013;1:168-175.
40   Radich JP, Kopecky KJ, Appelbaum FR, et al. A randomized trial of dasatinib 100 mg versus
      imatinib 400 mg in newly diagnosed chronic-phase chronic myeloid leukemia. *Blood*.
      2012;120:3898-3905.
41   Baccarani M, Deininger MW, Rosti G, et al. European LeukemiaNet recommendations for the
      management of chronic myeloid leukaemia: *Blood*. 2013;122:872-884.
42   Hughes TP, Hochhaus A, Branford S, et al. Long-term prognostic significance of early
      molecular response to imatinib in newly diagnosed chronic myeloid leukemia: an
      analysis from the International Randomized Study of Interferon and STI571 (IRIS). *Blood*.
      2010;116:3758-3765.
43   Hughes TP, Saglio G, Kantarjian HM, et al. Early molecular response predicts outcomes in
      patients with chronic myeloid leukemia in chronic phase treated with frontline nilotinib or
      imatinib. *Blood*. 2014;123:1353-1360.
44   Hehlmann R, Lauseker M, Jung-Munkwitz S, et al. Tolerability-adapted imatinib 800 mg/d
      versus 400 mg/d versus 400 mg/d plus interferon-α in newly diagnosed chronic myeloid
      leukemia. *J Clin Oncol*. 2011;29:1634-1642.
45   Johnson-Ansah H, Guilhot J, Rousselot P, et al. Tolerability and efficacy of pegylated
      interferon-α-2a in combination with imatinib for patients with chronic-phase chronic
      myeloid leukemia. *Cancer*. 2013;119:4284-4289.

Chapter 5

Challenges of treatment: tyrosine kinase inhibitor-resistant chronic myeloid leukemia

Mechanisms of resistance

Resistance to tyrosine kinase inhibitors (TKIs) can be defined on the basis of its time of onset. Primary resistance is a failure to achieve a significant therapeutic response, whereas secondary or acquired resistance is the progressive reappearance of the leukemic clone after an initial response to the drug. The frequency of primary resistance is dependent on the goals of therapy, but failure to achieve a hematological response is seen in <2% of patients and failure to achieve at least a major cytogenetic response (MCyR) in <10% of patients [1].

When confronted with a patient who is not responding, or ceases to respond to a TKI, the first question that should be asked is whether the drug is, in fact, being taken as prescribed. Lack of adherence to oral therapy for chronic diseases is a well-recognized problem, even among patients with a potentially fatal disease, such as cancer. It has been well documented that compliance to therapy is one of the major factors in determining the achievement of an adequate molecular response in patients being treated long term with imatinib [2,3]. Thus, before embarking on a series of expensive, and sometimes complex, laboratory tests to investigate whether the TKI is exerting its kinase inhibition effect, one has to ascertain that the cells are really being exposed to the drug.

© Springer International Publishing Switzerland 2014
T.P. Hughes et al., *Handbook of Chronic Myeloid Leukemia*,
DOI 10.1007/978-3-319-08350-6_5

BCR–ABL-dependent resistance

The development of point mutations in the *ABL* kinase domain is the most frequent mechanism of acquired resistance, but it is rare in patients who fail to show any response to the drug. It is important to emphasize that mutations are not induced by the drug, but rather, as with antibiotic resistance in bacteria, arise through a process whereby rare pre-existing mutant clones are self-selected due to their capacity to survive and expand in the presence of the drug, thus gradually outgrowing drug-sensitive cells.

Mutations are broadly categorized into four groups: (1) those that directly impair the TKI binding; (2) those within the ATP binding site; (3) those within the activation loop, preventing the kinase from achieving the conformation required for TKI binding; and (4) those within the catalytic domain [4] (Figure 5.1).

Thus far, close to 100 different point mutations leading to substitution of approximately 50 amino acids in the *ABL* kinase domain have been isolated from chronic myeloid leukemia (CML) patients resistant to imatinib [5] (Figure 5.1). The degree of imatinib resistance varies between mutations. For example, the *E255K, E255V,* and *T315I* mutations lead to a greater than 200-fold decrease in biochemical sensitivity to imatinib and correspondingly low levels of cellular sensitivity to the drug, while other mutations such as *F311L, F359V, V379I,* and *L387M* confer less than a threefold decrease in sensitivity [6]. These different degrees of sensitivity to imatinib are predicted to affect prognosis and response to treatment [7].

Approximately half of the patients who commence a second-generation TKI after failing imatinib therapy have detectable imatinib-resistant *BCR–ABL* mutations. Some of these mutants are also resistant to the newer inhibitors and, therefore, the identification of the type of amino acid substitution is of paramount importance before changing TKI therapy [8] (Figure 5.2).

Thus, the *V299L* and *F317L* mutations are predominantly associated with dasatinib failure; CML patients with leukemic clones that have these two mutants should therefore be treated with nilotinib [8]. Conversely, the finding of *F359V/C, Y253H,* or *E255K/V* at the decision point for a second-generation TKI is a strong recommendation for choosing dasatinib, as clones harboring these mutants are seldom responsive to nilotinib [8].

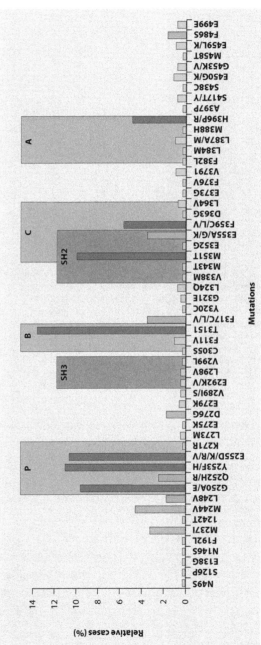

Figure 5.1 Relative incidence of mutations in clinical practice. Incidence of reported mutations within the kinase domain by percentage of total. The seven most frequent mutations are depicted in red and the following eight in blue; mutations shown in green have been reported in less than 2% of clinical resistance cases. Specific regions of the kinase domain are indicated as P-loop or ATP-binding site (P), imatinib-binding site (B), catalytic domain (C), and activation loop (A). Also shown as SH2 and SH3 are the contact regions with SH2 and SH3 domain-containing proteins. Adapted with permission from © Elsevier, 2007. All rights reserved. Apperley [4]. Adapted with permission from © Elsevier, 2014. All rights reserved. Soverini et al [5].

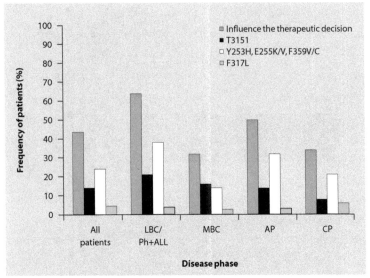

Figure 5.2 Frequency of patients with mutations where one or more of their mutations would influence the therapeutic decision. The frequency of detection of kinase domain mutations that are known to be resistant to either dasatinib or nilotinib or both drugs in CML patients receiving imatinib, expressed as a percentage of all patients with mutations detected. Results are shown according to the phase of disease when the patients first received imatinib therapy. ALL, acute lymphocytic leukemia; AP, accelerated phase; CP, chronic phase; LBC, lymphoid blast crisis; MBC, myeloid blast crisis; Ph, Philadelphia. Reproduced with permission from © American Society of Hematology, 2009. All rights reserved. Branford et al [8].

Overexpression of the BCR–ABL protein due to amplification of the *BCR–ABL* gene leads to resistance by increasing the amount of target protein needed to be inhibited by the therapeutic dose of the drug. It has been reported in a relatively small proportion of patients [4,9]. However, resistance due to BCR–ABL overexpression might be more frequent than genetic amplification. Cells expressing a high level of *BCR–ABL* have been observed to be far less sensitive to TKIs and develop resistant mutant subclones more rapidly than cells with low *BCR–ABL* expression levels [10,11]. This is probably related to the exacerbation of genomic instability by increased amounts of *BCR–ABL*, with a higher propensity to develop mutations anywhere in the genome, including the *BCR–ABL* kinase domain [10,12–14].

BCR–ABL-independent resistance

Mechanisms that lead to resistance independently of *BCR–ABL* are not so well understood, and some observations have not been reproduced by different investigators. They include defects in drug transport in and out of the leukemic cells, and activation of oncogenic pathways downstream of *BCR–ABL*.

Imatinib and other TKIs have been demonstrated to be substrates of P-glycoprotein (Pgp), the multi-drug resistance protein encoded by the *ABCB1* gene, as well as of *BRCP1*, encoded by the related *ABCG2* gene [15–18]. The intracellular levels of imatinib were shown to be significantly lower in Pgp-expressing cells [19–22]. However, clinical studies have failed to find a consistent association, and inhibition of Pgp does not seem to enhance the effect of imatinib against *BCR–ABL* activity [23–25]. Furthermore, recent studies showed that *ABCB1* and *ABCG2* seem to have a minimal functional role in the transport of imatinib in primary CML CD34+ cells, despite the high mRNA expression of these efflux pumps in CML progenitors [26,27].

The human organic cation transporter 1 (OCT-1) mediates the active transport of imatinib into cells, and inhibition of OCT-1 decreases the intracellular concentration of imatinib [28]. Some studies have shown that the functional activity at baseline, but not the expression level of the OCT-1 protein, is predictive of long-term outcome in patients with chronic phase CML treated with imatinib [29,30]. By contrast, recent data from other investigators [2,31] supported initial reports [23,24] showing that the level of OCT-1 transcripts in mononuclear cells (MNCs) have a significant prognostic value for response in CML. The reasons for such discrepancy in establishing the value of measuring OCT-1 mRNA levels as a prognostic marker are not apparent. Unlike imatinib, the intracellular concentrations of dasatinib and nilotinib are not significantly affected by OCT-1 activity, as their cellular influx is predominantly passive [22,32,33].

Overexpression and *BCR–ABL*-independent activation of Lyn, a phospho-serine/threonine rich sequence (SRC) kinase, was described in cells from CML patients who were resistant to imatinib [34,35] and nilotinib [36]. A polymorphic heterozygote deletion of the BCL-2-interacting mediator of cell death (*BIM*) pro-apoptotic gene, with a 12% allelic frequency in the Asian population but rare in Caucasians, was shown to mediate intrinsic resistance and inferior response to TKIs – the deletion was found in 29% of Asian patients resistant to imatinib, but in only 8% of those with a good response to the drug [37].

Several proteomics and microarray-based studies have disclosed genes, which may be over or underexpressed in imatinib-resistant cells as compared with their sensitive counterparts [38–40]. Many of these encode proteins involved in signal transduction and/or transcriptional regulation, which could, in principle, be associated with the development of resistance to imatinib independently of *BCR–ABL* kinase activity. However, there is as yet no conclusive functional evidence that any of these candidate proteins identified by microarray screenings are indeed causally responsible for clinical resistance in CML patients. This type of profiling may be more useful in identifying patterns of gene expression that may be predictive of poor response (primary resistance) to imatinib, as shown by different groups [41,42].

Another important fact is that, in vivo, CML cells treated with TKI are in a cytokine-rich environment. For this reason, inhibition of cytokine signaling pathways that directly or indirectly reinforce the oncogenic effect of *BCR–ABL* (eg, Janus kinase 2 [JAK2] and interleukin 3 [IL-3]) may restore the sensitivity of CML progenitors to TKI doses that had originally proven ineffective [43–45].

Lately, attention has been focused on the fact that CML leukemic stem cells are resistant to TKI-induced apoptosis, even when intracellular levels of the individual TKI are similar to those obtained in more mature CML cells [46–49]. Furthermore, it has been shown that, in vitro, these cells survive in spite of nearly complete inhibition of *BCR–ABL* kinase activity by the TKIs, suggesting that their primary resistance is *BCR–ABL* kinase-independent [50,51]. Thus, it is possible, although not yet demonstrated, that a pool of such cells may remain dormant as a residual, highly resistant population of CML stem cells in vivo, with the capacity to repopulate the leukemic clone, even in patients with a deep molecular response. This phenomenon is being intensively investigated, in the search for genes and proteins that may be linked to the apparently *BCR–ABL*-independent resistance mechanism in CML stem cells.

Therapeutic options for patients who fail frontline therapy

Under the revised European Leukemia Net (ELN) guidelines [52] a response that is not optimal but not poor enough to qualify as failure is categorized as a 'warning'. This has similar implications to the previously defined 'suboptimal' group. Long-term outcomes are probably inferior but there is no compelling evidence that a change in therapy will be beneficial. Many of these patients will eventually develop imatinib failure so they need to be closely observed. There is a general consensus [52] that patients who fail imatinib therapy should switch without hesitation to either nilotinib or dasatinib. The choice should be guided by the mutation profile, if relevant, and the comorbidities of the patient. Certain kinase domain mutations are unlikely to respond to nilotinib and a distinct set of mutations are unlikely to respond to dasatinib. Fortunately, the only mutation that is unlikely to respond to either dasatinib or nilotinib is the *T315I* mutation. The frequency of one of these mutations being present is variable in the different phases of the disease but in the chronic phase this frequency is around 10% (Figure 5.2) [8].

The probability of achieving a good response to second-line therapy can be predicted, based on a few baseline variables [53,54]. One of the strongest predictors of response to second-line therapy is response to first-line therapy. In an MD Anderson study, 3-year event-free survival for patients who had achieved MCyR on imatinib before treatment failure was 67% after switching to second-line therapy compared with 30% in patients with no prior cytogenetic response to imatinib [54]. Furthermore the success of switching can be assessed quite early, based on the molecular response 3 months after switching [55]. Patients with >10% *BCR–ABL* after 3 months on second-line treatment have an extremely low probability of achieving a stable deep molecular response.

For patients who fail frontline nilotinib or dasatinib therapy the course of action is less clear. The salvage rate when switching from dasatinib to nilotinib or vice versa is relatively low. In the case of mutations that are clearly susceptible to the second-line drug, this may be an effective approach, but for most patients this approach is unlikely to achieve stable molecular response in the long term. By contrast, the Ponatinib Ph ALL and CML Evaluation trial (PACE) trial demonstrated that in the second-line and even in the third-line setting there was a reasonable expectation of response to ponatinib [56]. Ponatinib is an *ABL* inhibitor with SRC activity that is active against the *T315I* mutation as well as all other single-point mutations that have been studied.

Other tyrosine kinase inhibitors after failure of frontline therapy

Bosutinib

Bosutinib is a potent second-generation TKI that, as with dasatinib, also has SRC inhibitory activity. In the Bosutinib Efficacy and Safety in Chronic Myeloid LeukemiA (BELA) Phase III randomized study, bosutinib failed to demonstrate superior rates of CCyR compared with imatinib at 12 months in patients with newly diagnosed, chronic-phase CML [57]. However, the response and progression rates achieved with bosutinib were similar to those achieved with nilotinib and dasatinib in this setting [57]. Further studies may establish a place for bosutinib in the frontline setting. The safety profile of bosutinib is generally favorable, although gastrointestinal toxicity is common in the first few months of therapy. No long-term organ toxicity has been identified, but exposure to bosutinib has been quite limited to date. For the moment, it is registered in many countries as a second-line or third-line option. In a Phase II study, 23% of patients who were resistant to imatinib as well as either nilotinib or dasatinib achieved CCyR on bosutinib at 24 weeks. Discouragingly, only 24% of these patients remain on bosutinib long term in this study [58].

Ponatinib

Ponatinib is the only clinically available TKI that has activity against the *T315I* mutation. This mutation is resistant to all other available TKIs, so for patients with this mutation who do not have an option to proceed to an allograft, ponatinib represents the only opportunity to achieve molecular response and long-term disease control. However, its activity is not confined to the *T315I* mutant form of *BCR–ABL*. The Phase I and II (PACE) studies have demonstrated that a high proportion of patients resistant to two or more TKIs will achieve excellent responses to ponatinib [56]. Although patients with the *T315I* mutation had higher rates of response (MCyR rates of 70% in *T315I* patients versus 50% in other resistant or intolerant patients, median follow-up 11 months), a multivariate analysis found that younger age and higher dose intensity were the most significant predictors of response, not the presence of the *T315I* mutation. A potential drawback of using ponatinib is the toxicity profile. Pancreatitis can be a significant problem for some patients but rarely leads to drug cessation. More importantly a significant association with vascular events has recently been recognized with rates of arterial and venous vascular events of over 20% [56]. Concern about the increasing rate of vascular events in the US led the US Food and Drug Administration (FDA) to withdraw ponatinib temporarily from the market. Recently it has become available again but under a more restricted indication. It is now indicated for any patient with a *T315I* mutation and for other patients where no other TKI is indicated. Significant cerebrovascular events have been reported and venous as well as arterial thromboses have been observed. Given this risk profile, ponatinib should be reserved for patients where no other TKI is likely to be effective and safe. Its use should be restricted in patients with previous vascular events or diabetes where the risk of a new vascular event is high – these patients should be fully informed about the risks involved. Ponatinib should also be used at the lowest dose possible that can maintain an adequate response. There is some emerging evidence that lower doses are associated with a lower risk of vascular events and that these modified doses can still maintain molecular responses in many cases [59]. Clearly the role of ponatinib is under review as these new toxicity data are analyzed more closely and the recommendations described here may be subject to revision.

Allogeneic stem cell transplantation
When should a donor search be initiated?
It is generally not cost effective to conduct tissue typing studies to look for potentially suitable donors in chronic phase CML patients at diagnosis. The vast majority will never be considered for an allograft. In the event of failure of TKI therapy, in patients who are potential candidates for

an allograft, it is probably cost effective to proceed with a donor search just in case the second-line therapy is unsuccessful or there is evidence of disease transformation where any delay due to donor searching issues would be highly undesirable.

When is it the right option?

An allograft should not be considered as a frontline option for any CML patient who is in chronic phase, including children. However, an allograft should still be considered in some patients who fail frontline therapy. With the availability of ponatinib, there has been a need to modify the indications for allogeneic transplantation in CML. Previously, patients who developed the *T315I* mutation were considered to be immediately eligible for an allograft because none of the available TKIs had any activity against this mutation. Now ponatinib may be a reasonable choice for some of these patients (with the important provisos discussed above). Who, then, should receive an allograft for CML today? There are two categories: (1) any patient who presents in blast crisis or progresses to accelerated phase or blast crisis on therapy should be assessed for an allograft without delay and ideally proceed to an allograft as soon as chronic phase can be re-established [60]; and (2) Patients who remain in the chronic phase but have failed a second-generation TKI and are not eligible for ponatinib or have failed a trial of ponatinib therapy [61,62].

Outcomes of allografts for patients who have developed TKI resistance but remain in the chronic phase are generally favorable. Myeloablative or reduced intensity conditioning have been used in this setting with both achieving similar outcomes. T-cell depletion of the donor stem cells is not usually applied because of the much higher risk of disease relapse in this setting.

References

1   Hochhaus A, O'Brien SG, Guilhot F, et al. Six-year follow-up of patients receiving imatinib for the first-line treatment of chronic myeloid leukemia. *Leukemia.* 2009;23:1054-1061.
2   Marin D, Bazeos A, Mahon FX, et al. Adherence is the critical factor for achieving molecular responses in patients with chronic myeloid leukemia who achieve complete cytogenetic responses on imatinib. *J Clin Oncol.* 2010;28:2381-2388.
3   Ibrahim AR, Eliasson L, Apperley JF, et al. Poor adherence is the main reason for loss of CCyR and imatinib failure for CML patients on long term therapy. *Blood.* 2011;117:3733-3736.

4   Apperley JF. Part I: mechanisms of resistance to imatinib in chronic myeloid leukaemia. *Lancet Oncol.* 2007;8:1018-1029.

5   Soverini S, Branford S, Nicolini FE et al. Implications of BCR-ABL1 kinase domain-mediated resistance in chronic myeloid leukemia. *Leuk Res.* 2014;38:10-20.

6   Corbin AS, Rosee PL, Stoffregen EP, Druker BJ, Deininger MW. Several Bcr-Abl kinase domain mutants associated with imatinib mesylate resistance remain sensitive to imatinib. *Blood.* 2003;101:4611-4614.

7   Jabbour E, Soverini S. Understanding the role of mutations in therapeutic decision making for chronic myeloid leukemia. *Semin Hematol.* 2009;46:S22-S26.

8   Branford S, Melo JV, Hughes TP. Selecting optimal second-line tyrosine kinase inhibitor therapy for chronic myeloid leukemia patients after imatinib failure: does the BCR-ABL mutation status really matter? *Blood.* 2009;114:5426-5435.

9   Gambacorti-Passerini CB, Gunby RH, Piazza R, Galietta A, Rostagno R, Scapozza L. Molecular mechanisms of resistance to imatinib in Philadelphia-chromosome-positive leukaemias. *Lancet Oncol.* 2003;4:75-85.

10   Barnes DJ, Palaiologou D, Panousopoulou E, et al. Bcr-Abl expression levels determine the rate of development of resistance to imatinib mesylate in chronic myeloid leukemia. *Cancer Res.* 2005;65:8912-8919.

11   Tang C, Schafranek L, Watkins DB, et al. Tyrosine kinase inhibitor resistance in chronic myeloid leukemia cell lines: investigating resistance pathways. *Leuk Lymphoma.* 2011;52:2139-2147.

12   Koptyra M, Cramer K, Slupianek A, Richardson C, Skorski T. BCR/ABL promotes accumulation of chromosomal aberrations induced by oxidative and genotoxic stress. *Leukemia.* 2008;22:1969-1972.

13   Cramer K, Nieborowska-Skorska M, Koptyra M, et al. BCR/ABL and other kinases from chronic myeloproliferative disorders stimulate single-strand annealing, an unfaithful DNA double-strand break repair. *Cancer Res.* 2008;68:6884-6888.

14   Yuan H, Wang Z, Gao C, et al. BCR-ABL gene expression is required for its mutations in a novel KCL-22 cell culture model for acquired resistance of chronic myelogenous leukemia. *J Biol Chem.* 2010;285:5085-5096.

15   Burger H, van Tol H, Boersma AW, et al. Imatinib mesylate (STI571) is a substrate for the breast cancer resistance protein (BCRP)/ABCG2 drug pump. *Blood.* 2004;104:2940-2942.

16   Houghton PJ, Germain GS, Harwood FC, et al. Imatinib mesylate is a potent inhibitor of the ABCG2 (BCRP) transporter and reverses resistance to topotecan and SN-38 in vitro. *Cancer Res.* 2004;64:2333-2337.

17   Burger H, van Tol H, Brok M, et al. Chronic imatinib mesylate exposure leads to reduced intracellular drug accumulation by induction of the ABCG2 (BCRP) and ABCB1 (MDR1) drug transport pumps. *Cancer Biol Ther.* 2005;4:747-752.

18   Jordanides NE, Jorgensen HG, Holyoake TL, Mountford JC. Functional ABCG2 is overexpressed on primary CML CD34+ cells and is inhibited by imatinib mesylate. *Blood.* 2006;108:1370-1373.

19   Hegedus T, Orfi L, Seprodi A, Varadi A, Sarkadi B, Keri G. Interaction of tyrosine kinase inhibitors with the human multidrug transporter proteins, MDR1 and MRP1. *Biochim Biophys Acta.* 2002;1587:318-325.

20   Jiang X, Zhao Y, Smith C et al. Chronic myeloid leukemia stem cells possess multiple unique features of resistance to BCR-ABL targeted therapies. *Leukemia.* 2007;21:926-935.

21   Giannoudis A, Davies A, Lucas CM, Harris RJ, Pirmohamed M, Clark RE. Effective dasatinib uptake may occur without human organic cation transporter 1 (hOCT1): implications for the treatment of imatinib-resistant chronic myeloid leukemia. *Blood.* 2008;112:3348-3354.

22   Hiwase DK, Saunders V, Hewett D, et al. Dasatinib cellular uptake and efflux in chronic myeloid leukemia cells: therapeutic implications. *Clin Cancer Res.* 2008;14:3881-3888.

23   Crossman LC, Druker BJ, Deininger MW, Pirmohamed M, Wang L, Clark RE. hOCT 1 and resistance to imatinib. *Blood.* 2005;106:1133-1134.

24   Wang L, Giannoudis A, Lane S, Williamson P, Pirmohamed M, Clark RE. Expression of the uptake drug transporter hOCT1 is an important clinical determinant of the response to imatinib in chronic myeloid leukemia. *Clin Pharmacol Ther.* 2008;83:258-264.

25   Hatziieremia S, Jordanides NE, Holyoake TL, Mountford JC, Jorgensen HG. Inhibition of MDR1 does not sensitize primitive chronic myeloid leukemia CD34+ cells to imatinib. *Exp Hematol.* 2009;37:692-700.

26   Engler JR, Frede A, Saunders VA, Zannettino AC, Hughes TP, White DL. Chronic myeloid leukemia CD34+ cells have reduced uptake of imatinib due to low OCT-1 activity. *Leukemia.* 2010;24:765-770.

27   Eadie LN, Hughes TP, White DL. Interaction of the efflux transporters ABCB1 and ABCG2 with imatinib, nilotinib, and dasatinib. *Clin Pharmacol Ther.* 2014;95:294-306.

28   Thomas J, Wang L, Clark RE, Pirmohamed M. Active transport of imatinib into and out of cells: implications for drug resistance. *Blood.* 2004;104:3739-3745.

29   White DL, Saunders VA, Dang P, et al. Most CML patients who have a suboptimal response to imatinib have low OCT-1 activity: higher doses of imatinib may overcome the negative impact of low OCT-1 activity. *Blood.* 2007;110:4064-4072.

30   White DL, Dang P, Engler J, et al. Functional activity of the OCT-1 protein is predictive of long-term outcome in patients with chronic-phase chronic myeloid leukemia treated with imatinib. *J Clin Oncol.* 2010;28:2761-2767.

31   Bazeos A, Marin D, Reid AG, et al. hOCT1 transcript levels and single nucleotide polymorphisms as predictive factors for response to imatinib in chronic myeloid leukemia. *Leukemia.* 2010;24:1243-1245.

32   Davies A, Jordanides NE, Giannoudis A, et al. Nilotinib concentration in cell lines and primary CD34(+) chronic myeloid leukemia cells is not mediated by active uptake or efflux by major drug transporters. *Leukemia.* 2009;23:1999-2006.

33   Eadie L, Hughes TP, White DL. Nilotinib does not significantly reduce imatinib OCT-1 activity in either cell lines or primary CML cells. *Leukemia.* 2010;24:855-857.

34   Donato NJ, Wu JY, Stapley J, et al. BCR-ABL independence and LYN kinase overexpression in chronic myelogenous leukemia cells selected for resistance to STI571. *Blood.* 2003;101:690-698.

35   Dai Y, Rahmani M, Corey SJ, Dent P, Grant S. A Bcr/Abl-independent, Lyn-dependent form of imatinib mesylate (STI-571) resistance is associated with altered expression of Bcl-2. *J Biol Chem.* 2004;279:34227-34239.

36   Mahon FX, Hayette S, Lagarde V, et al. Evidence that resistance to nilotinib may be due to BCR-ABL, Pgp, or Src kinase overexpression. *Cancer Res.* 2008;68:9809-9816.

37   Ng KP, Hillmer AM, Chuah CT, et al. A common BIM deletion polymorphism mediates intrinsic resistance and inferior responses to tyrosine kinase inhibitors in cancer. *Nat Med.* 2012;18:521-528.

38   Tipping AJ, Deininger MW, Goldman JM, Melo JV. Comparative gene expression profile of chronic myeloid leukemia cells innately resistant to imatinib mesylate. *Exp Hematol.* 2003;31:1073-1080.

39   Frank O, Brors B, Fabarius A, et al. Gene expression signature of primary imatinib-resistant chronic myeloid leukemia patients. *Leukemia.* 2006;20:1400-1407.

40   Grosso S, Puissant A, Dufies M, et al. Gene expression profiling of imatinib and PD166326-resistant CML cell lines identifies Fyn as a gene associated with resistance to BCR-ABL inhibitors. *Mol Cancer Ther.* 2009;8:1924-1933.

41   McWeeney SK, Pemberton LC, Loriaux MM, et al. A gene expression signature of CD34+ cells to predict major cytogenetic response in chronic-phase chronic myeloid leukemia patients treated with imatinib. *Blood.* 2010;115:315-325.

42   de Lavallade H, Finetti P, Carbuccia N, et al. A gene expression signature of primary resistance to imatinib in chronic myeloid leukemia. *Leuk Res.* 2010;34:254-257.

43   Hiwase DK, White DL, Powell JA et al. Blocking cytokine signaling along with intense Bcr-Abl kinase inhibition induces apoptosis in primary CML progenitors. *Leukemia.* 2010;24:771-778.

44 Shah NP, Kasap C, Weier C, et al. Transient potent BCR-ABL inhibition is sufficient to commit chronic myeloid leukemia cells irreversibly to apoptosis. *Cancer Cell.* 2008;14:485-493.

45 Nievergall E, Ramshaw HS, Yong AS, et al. Monoclonal antibody targeting of IL-3 receptor alpha with CSL362 effectively depletes CML progenitor and stem cells. *Blood.* 2014;123:1218-1228.

46 Holtz MS, Forman SJ, Bhatia R. Nonproliferating CML CD34+ progenitors are resistant to apoptosis induced by a wide range of proapoptotic stimuli. *Leukemia.* 2005;19:1034-1041.

47 Copland M, Hamilton A, Elrick LJ, et al. Dasatinib (BMS-354825) targets an earlier progenitor population than imatinib in primary CML but does not eliminate the quiescent fraction. *Blood.* 2006;107:4532-4539.

48 Jorgensen HG, Allan EK, Jordanides NE, Mountford JC, Holyoake TL. Nilotinib exerts equipotent anti-proliferative effects to imatinib and does not induce apoptosis in CD34+ CML cells. *Blood.* 2007;4016-4019.

49 Konig H, Holtz M, Modi H, et al. Enhanced BCR-ABL kinase inhibition does not result in increased inhibition of downstream signaling pathways or increased growth suppression in CML progenitors. *Leukemia.* 2008;22:748-755.

50 Corbin AS, Agarwal A, Loriaux M, Cortes J, Deininger MW, Druker BJ. Human chronic myeloid leukemia stem cells are insensitive to imatinib despite inhibition of BCR-ABL activity. *J Clin Invest.* 2011;121:396-409.

51 Hamilton A, Helgason GV, Schemionek M et al. Chronic myeloid leukemia stem cells are not dependent on Bcr-Abl kinase activity for their survival. *Blood.* 2012;119:1501-1510.

52 Baccarani M, Deininger MW, Rosti G, et al. European LeukemiaNet recommendations for the management of chronic myeloid leukemia: 2013. *Blood.* 2013;122:872-884.

53 Milojkovic D, Nicholson E, Apperley JF, et al. Early prediction of success or failure of treatment with second-generation tyrosine kinase inhibitors in patients with chronic myeloid leukemia. *Haematologica.* 2010;95:224-231.

54 Jabbour E, le Coutre PD, Cortes J, et al. Prediction of outcomes in patients with Ph+ chronic myeloid leukemia in chronic phase treated with nilotinib after imatinib resistance/intolerance. *Leukemia.* 2013;27:907-913.

55 Branford S, Kim DW, Soverini S, et al. Initial molecular response at 3 months may predict both response and event-free survival at 24 months in imatinib-resistant or -intolerant patients with Philadelphia chromosome-positive chronic myeloid leukemia in chronic phase treated with nilotinib. *J Clin Oncol.* 2012;30:4323-4329.

56 Cortes JE, Kim DW, Pinilla-Ibarz J, et al. A phase 2 trial of ponatinib in Philadelphia chromosome-positive leukemias. *N Engl J Med.* 2013;369:1783-1796.

57 Cortes JE, Kim DW, Kantarjian HM, et al. Bosutinib versus imatinib in newly diagnosed chronic-phase chronic myeloid leukemia: results from the BELA trial. *J Clin Oncol.* 2012;30:3486-3492.

58 Cortes JE, Kantarjian HM, Brummendorf TH, et al. Safety and efficacy of bosutinib (SKI-606) in chronic phase Philadelphia chromosome-positive chronic myeloid leukemia patients with resistance or intolerance to imatinib. *Blood.* 2011;118:4567-4576.

59 Hochaus A, Pinilla-Ibarz J, Kim D-W, et al. Clinical impact of dose modification and dose intensity on response to ponatinib (PON) in patients (pts) with Philadelphia chromosome-positive (Ph+) leukemias. *J Clin Oncol;* ASCO Annual Meeting Abstracts. 2014;32:(suppl)7084.

60 Hehlmann R. How I treat CML blast crisis. *Blood.* 2012;120:737-747.

61 Khoury HJ, Kukreja M, Goldman JM, et al. Prognostic factors for outcomes in allogeneic transplantation for CML in the imatinib era: a CIBMTR analysis. *Bone Marrow Transplant.* 2012;47:810-816.

62 Saussele S, Lauseker M, Gratwohl A, et al. Allogeneic hematopoietic stem cell transplantation (allo SCT) for chronic myeloid leukemia in the imatinib era: evaluation of its impact within a subgroup of the randomized German CML Study IV. *Blood.* 2010;115:1880-1885.

CPSIA information can be obtained
at www.ICGtesting.com
Printed in the USA
BVHW010221080819
555398BV00005B/90/P

9 783319 083490